SUCCESSFUL SURGERY AND HEALING:

A PRACTICAL GUIDE
FOR PATIENTS, CAREGIVERS AND ADVOCATES

LORI L. MERTZ

JUST BEE PUBLISHING
SALT LAKE CITY, UTAH

Just Bee Publishing
P.O. Box 526376
Salt Lake City, Utah 84152
WWW.LORIMERTZ.COM

Book cover design by Josh Yamamoto.
Book layout by BOOKDESIGNTEMPLATES.COM.
Images used with permission.

Ordering Information:
Just Bee publications may be ordered through booksellers or by contacting publisher at the address above. Special discounts may be available on quantity purchases by corporations, associations, schools, non-profits and others. For details, contact the "Special Sales Department" at the address above.

Successful Surgery and Healing: A Practical Guide For Patients, Caregivers and Advocates / Lori L. Mertz. —1st ed.
ISBN 978-0-6158462-4-8

Printed in the United States of America

This book is dedicated to you, the reader.
This information is for you.
You can do this!

And, to the amazing doctors I've been fortunate to have on my journey.
Thank you for all you've shared and taught me; I am so grateful!
May the cycle continue and others benefit from
the kindnesses and respect you showed me.

All reasonable effort has been made to ensure the accuracy of the information in this book. This book contains informational materials and opinions and is intended for educational purposes. The information contained herewith is not meant to treat, diagnose, prescribe or cure any ailment and is not intended as a substitute for professional medical care. Only your doctor can diagnose and treat a medical problem. Consult your doctor before you start, stop or change anything that has been previously prescribed or before following any advice. Be aware, certain remedies are unsuitable for individuals with certain medical ailments. The Author and Publisher shall not be liable for any damages allegedly arising from the information in this book. The opinions expressed in this book are the Author's alone.

Having said that, **become a full and active partner in your medical care**. Ask questions about doctor-recommended treatments, plans, procedures, therapies and prescribed medicines until you obtain satisfactory answers and are completely comfortable. Get second opinions. Educate yourself. Do your own research and ask more questions.

Contents

PART II: IF YOU HAVE TIME TO PLAN AND PREPARE

Foreword

You hold in your hands the final product of a lot of dedicated time and effort. It is the result of research, direct experience and a thorough education resulting from the author's personal experiences with surgery and recovery and what she learned along the way.

I first met Lori Mertz in 1998. She came to see me as a patient to help her figure out why she was fatigued. Prior to seeing me Lori had undergone open-heart surgery, knee surgery and an appendectomy. With my help, as her primary care physician, Lori conquered her fatigue. Subsequently, we worked together as she recovered from a traumatic brain injury and later back surgery, pulling from the frontiers of both allopathic and complementary medicine.

Lori is an enthusiastic, interesting, diligent, proactive patient and willing to learn. She would follow the regimens we created and return with a list of what was and was not working and questions directed at continually clarifying and refining her experiences. It is an ongoing education. Out of that education and her ample personal experiences has come this book.

Although I'm a family practice physician, I rarely find myself in the hospital. As an integrative medicine physician for over 25 years, my work is focused on how to restore people to optimal health. What became apparent as this book came into being is that the principles for the creation of health apply equally to those who come to my wellness center and to those who find themselves in a hospital and recovering from surgery. Knowing how hard it is to distill complex technical information in a way that it remains easy to understand and completely intact, I assisted Lori by carefully reviewing the medical information included for accuracy and accessibility.

With millions of people undergoing surgery each year, *Successful Surgery and Healing* is a timely compilation designed to allow patients to participate in their own care. It supports patients and the people who love them through the experience. It includes what everyone needs to know as they prepare for, recover and heal from surgery. It encompasses everything from the medical to the practical to the legal aspects surrounding surgery.

With her willingness and open heart, Lori and *Successful Surgery and Healing* are there for those seeking a surgical guide and a successful surgical experience. *Successful Surgery and Healing* answers the question "What do I need to know?" for those who don't know what they don't know. It provides support, structure and tools.

This book is also for anyone in the medical and caregiving fields. Surgeons should give each patient a copy of this book as part of their pre-surgery care!

Todd A. Mangum, M.D.
Director, Web of Life Wellness Center

Introduction

"Wouldn't you agree that a well-informed,
well-prepared patient is more relaxed and positive and
has a better post-surgical outcome?"

Every doctor I've posed this question to has answered the same. Their answer is always a resounding "Yes!" It's the reason I wrote this book.

∎ ∎ ∎

SURGERY HAPPENS

Accidents. Injury. Illness. They aren't planned, but happen at some point to ourselves and the people we know. While I don't wish these experiences on anyone, because of what I've been through in my lifetime—a seemingly unusual number of surgeries—I have learned a great deal and have a unique perspective into the surgical process, healing and recovery. I'm not writing this book because I'm a doctor, but because I am a successful patient. And you can be one, too!

There are two kinds of surgery: planned and unplanned (or emergency). Planned surgery is surgery that does not involve a medical emergency and does not need to be performed immediately. Unplanned surgery arises from an accident or other emergency. It is surgery that must be performed immediately or within a day or two.

No matter where you are in the surgical process—beginning, middle or end—there is information here for you. This book is for everyone: Those who live alone, couples and families. It's also for caretakers, advocates, friends and care providers. The ideas, checklists, templates and worksheets contained within are for anyone preparing for or recovering from surgery, whether planned or unplanned.

While your present circumstance may feel daunting or overwhelming,
know that you can do this!

To each reader, may this material help and support you on your journey through surgery and healing, to your state of optimum health and wellness.

A LITTLE ABOUT ME...

I have had both planned and unplanned emergency surgery; in fact, several of each between the ages of 19 to 42.

PLANNED SURGERY	UNPLANNED EMERGENCY SURGERY & ACCIDENTS
Open-heart surgery, age 21	Partially severed left Achilles tendon, age 19
Left knee reconstruction, age 24	Appendectomy, age 32
Right knee reconstruction, age 37	Traumatic brain injury (TBI), age 34
Micro-lumbar-discectomy, age 42	

The surgeries I've undergone were the result of a congenital defect (open-heart surgery), an acute medical emergency (bursting appendix), sports-related injuries (knees) and accidents (TBI from a bike accident and a partially severed Achilles tendon caused by a heavy steel door slamming on my heel).

I came upon my particular expertise surrounding surgery honestly, reluctantly and very much by accident—literally and figuratively.

The surgeries I had took place in various cities across the country depending on where I was living at the time (Boston, Salt Lake City, Newport Beach); sometimes near family and sometimes very far away. I shot from the hip and did the best I could, but even when I had time to plan, I often wasn't really prepared for what took place. Being a single adult who was living alone added a particular kind of challenge and twist to both planned and unplanned surgeries and injuries alike.

WHAT I'VE LEARNED OVER THE YEARS

I have learned that, first and foremost, we need each other for help and support. I learned what an advocate is and why having one is so important and valuable. I learned a lot about patience and what it really means. I learned that with unplanned emergency surgery you lose a lot of control; you don't get to pick your doctor or hospital or have time to get organized physically, mentally or emotionally. I learned that hospitals are for critical care and pain management, healing takes place at home. In a nutshell, I learned that when it comes to taking care of ourselves—body, mind, emotions and spirit—there is a lot to know.

When navigating surgery and healing, I found that not only is there a lot to know,
I didn't know what I didn't know.

My experiences could have undoubtedly been easier if I'd had more complete information about what to expect before, during and after surgery. Simple checklists (such as the ones provided inside) would have been very helpful in getting myself organized and creating structure. I wish I had known what kind of help to ask for. I wish I'd been more compassionate and patient with myself during the healing and recovery process; it's a journey, not a sprint. I wish I'd known then what I know now.

My education came full circle when I was 42 years old and required back surgery. One thing I was acutely aware of as I prepared was that I was going to need help and support.

Armed with a clear intention to be better prepared than before, I set out. What came of that intention is included in the pages that follow.

Start here and now and make this book your own. Borrow my questions. Use my checklists and templates.[i] Bookmark pages. Write in the margins and spaces provided. Take what works and discard the rest. There is no one way to prepare for or recover from surgery.

The right way is the way that works for you!

■ ■ ■

Here's what I believe and know for sure: you can absolutely do this! If you're unsure about that in this moment, hang in there and take it one step at a time. Be patient. Ask questions. Believe in yourself and in your body's innate healing abilities. I did it when I was sure I couldn't and you can too. It's amazing the inner strength each of us harbor.

"One of the good things about life's challenges:
You get to find out that you're capable of being far more than you ever thought possible."
Karen Salmansohn

However, we may not be aware of that incredible strength—or what we are capable of—until we are faced with a situation that causes us to tap into it. This was the case for me. Until I was faced with having to undergo open-heart surgery I would have never believed that I could do it and yet, I did. I found that same inner strength available to me after my head injury and when I had to undergo back surgery. It is always there when I've needed it and I absolutely know it's available to everyone.

---

[i] Each of the templates included at the end of this book are also available as free 8 ½" x 11" .docx and .pdf downloads at LORIMERTZ.COM/FREE-DOWNLOADS.HTML.

May the wisdom, stories and tools shared within (from doctors, nurses, physical therapists, patients, family members, advocates, caregivers and personal experience) empower and support you in having a successful surgical experience and on your journey to perfect health and wholeness.

PART I:

SURGERY. WHAT EVERYONE NEEDS TO KNOW—WHETHER SURGERY IS PLANNED OR UNPLANNED

1: GETTING STARTED

WHETHER YOU HAVE HAD PLANNED OR UNPLANNED SURGERY, START
HERE, WITH PART I.
Part I (pages 1-114) includes pertinent information that everyone needs
to know: getting an advocate; asking for help; creating a safe comfortable
environment; post-surgery information for healing and recovery at home.

**IF YOU HAVE TIME TO PLAN AND PREPARE, START WITH PART II, THEN RETURN
TO PART I.**

If timing allows, Part II (pages 117-168) contains valuable information on preparing for
surgery, getting organized ahead of time and what to expect. Start there, then go back
and read the valuable information contained in Part I.

THINGS TO REMEMBER:

- ☐ **There are no dumb or unimportant questions**. (Trust me, I've asked them all.)
- ☐ **Asking questions and getting satisfactory answers is your right** as a patient.
- ☐ **A good doctor should appreciate your questions** and be willing to explain information in a way you can understand, so you are prepared and feel safe.
- ☐ **Ask for help.**
- ☐ **You can do this.**

Get An Advocate

An advocate is an essential resource to have throughout
all stages of the surgical process: before surgery, at the hospital and after surgery.

■ ■ ■

WHAT IS AN ADVOCATE?

An advocate is a person who supports or argues for a cause or person. In a medical situation, an advocate is there on your behalf to take on a protective roll, someone you trust to have your back during an uncertain and possibly scary time. This person is your extra set of eyes and ears. Having an extra set of ears to hear important (often technical and overwhelming) information is extremely valuable.

An advocate can also be your voice when you can't or may be too afraid or too unwell to speak, such as during a doctor appointment or while you are in the hospital. As the patient, you might not feel up to talking or questioning things that don't make sense or that you need help with. This is where an advocate can step in and be helpful.

An advocate can also act as a gatekeeper, questioning recommended tests and procedures and checking prescribed medications that are being administered. They are also a great sounding board to bounce ideas, concerns and fears off as you navigate the surgery process, which can be complicated and confusing. Choose someone who lives in close proximity. An advocate that is far away may not be as effective as one who is physically present.

WHAT DOES AN ADVOCATE DO?

- **Assist you in having the experience you desire**. This person understands your wishes and is focused on you and your desired outcome; they are there just for you.
- **Attend pre- and post-surgery doctor's visits** with you. They can listen in and give you feedback on what they hear.
- **Help you sort through information and get clear** about what you want to do, if you feel overwhelmed.
- **Speak up on your behalf** when necessary.
- **Make sure you get appropriate care** in the hospital.
- **Check medications administered in the hospital**. This is especially important if you have serious or life-threatening allergies.
- **Write down post-surgery instructions** on your behalf. Following any kind of in- or out-patient surgery, you may be groggy from anesthesia or other medications. Knowing this, it's a good idea to have someone else—your advocate—take and review post-op surgical instructions with your doctor. Your advocate can then communicate these instructions to you later at home.

When I have had surgery or been in the hospital, I have usually been nervous, overwhelmed and sometimes in a lot of pain and on pain medication which kept me from being present and focused. An advocate is your person; someone who is present and focused on you and your care, when maybe you can't be. Thank you to my advocates!

It is estimated that in the U.S. there are approximately 550 deaths EACH DAY (200,000 a year) due to medical mistakes.[1] An advocate may help prevent a fatal error.

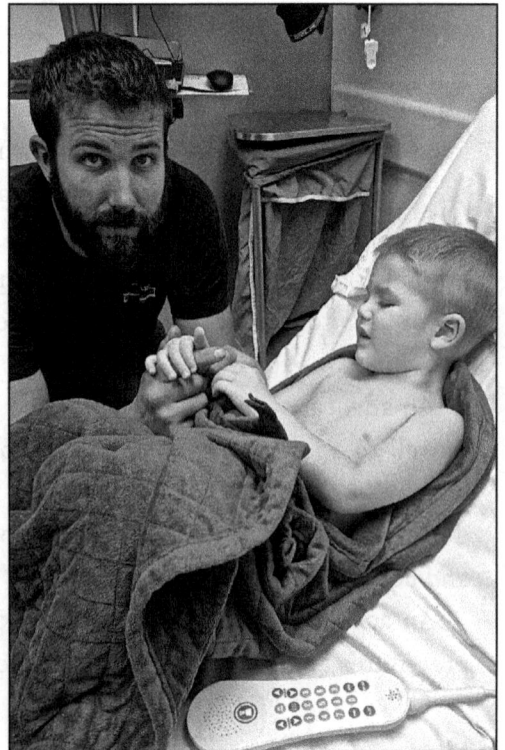

WHO SHOULD I CHOOSE AS MY ADVOCATE?

An advocate can be anyone you trust: a parent, sibling, relative, spouse, partner, significant other, friend, hired caregiver or combination thereof.

We naturally advocate and champion for our family and friends all the time. Children have a natural advocate in their parent or guardian, but due to distance and circumstance this relationship and support may not necessarily transition into adulthood. When facing important life-changing medical decisions we need our family and friends advocating and championing for us, making sure we receive proper medical care.

Note: In some cases, people assume their spouse will take on the role of an advocate, but this isn't always the case. Sometimes our best advocate may be someone else, someone not so close or emotionally involved.

TRAITS OF A GOOD ADVOCATE:

- Someone who is available and willing to be this resource.
- Someone in close proximity who you could call in the middle of the night, if necessary. Knowing your advocate is nearby may help you feel safe and more secure.
- Good active listening and communication skills; the ability to repeat back important points during meetings to make sure everyone is hearing and agreeing to the same thing.
- Inquisitive and proficient at clearly asking questions and expressing needs.
- Direct, but positive and courteous. (Aggressiveness can breed animosity.)
- Assertive and persistent, when necessary; willing to question information given.
- Willingness to speak up and fight for you or your care if necessary, when you can't speak or fight for yourself; be your voice if something's not going according to plan.

It will be up to you to determine which qualities are the most important for you to have in an advocate and to choose from the people you have available. My mother has been a fierce medical advocate for me on several occasions. Knowing she was keeping a watchful eye and taking care of business during medical crises made me feel safe and allowed me to relax, let go, rest and heal.

PREPARE YOUR ADVOCATE WITH YOUR WISHES

Arm your advocate with any pertinent documents you have that specifically address your wishes, should you become unable to communicate or do so yourself. If you don't already have an advance directive in place, now may be a good time to put pen to paper with your wishes in the event something unexpected occurs. You have the right to decide how you will be cared for, down to the last second, but unless it's written down it cannot be implemented on your behalf. If no such paperwork has been completed and you lose the capacity to make your own decisions, a doctor's only recourse is to consult with available *family* members. (See Appendix, pages 188-189 for information on documents recognized in the event of an emergency.)

WHAT IF I HAVE TO ADVOCATE FOR MYSELF?

If you have to advocate for yourself, use the same tips and tools described above. For example, if you have a serious or life-threatening allergy, you will need to remain vigilant and remind each doctor, nurse and attendant.

It may feel like you are constantly repeating yourself, but that's okay.

The single most important thing is you—your health, your safety and your well-being. If that means repeating yourself, so be it.

If you must advocate for yourself, know that you can do it. In fact, by reading this book, you are already advocating for yourself by becoming more informed and better prepared.

ADVOCATING FOR SOMEONE IN THE HOSPITAL

Here's how advocating for friends in the hospital can look: When a friend of mine was in the hospital, I would sit with him when his wife had to go to work. When his pain flared up, I encouraged him to buzz the nurse for pain medication (he had stoic tendencies). On one occasion, when the nurse hadn't arrived after 15 minutes, I encouraged him to buzz again. Since my friend was now in considerable pain and no one had showed up or told us when to expect the nurse we buzzed a third time. I also went to the nurse's station and inquired. When an unhelpful aide dismissed me, I calmly walked the halls until I found the nurse myself and made her aware of my friends situation and pain. Advocating for my friend meant taking matters into my own hands.

After the nurse arrived and administered the pain medication, I noted the time it was given, the name of the drug, the strength and dosage and when he would be able to have another dose if his pain returned. This information was also written on a white-board in his room and I texted it his wife so she would know what had taken place while she was away.

On the receiving end, after my head injury, when I was in the intensive care unit (ICU), my mother stayed with me for a week, checking and double-checking each medication that was administered and why.

Sometimes we need a ferocious advocate.

EVEN EXPERTS BLOW IT

Even with advanced degrees, sometimes doctors and institutions still don't get it right. Case in point: I have a friend who was in a car accident where she sustained some serious injuries, including a head injury. Years later, she went to a specialized head trauma clinic in Southern California to get information about her cognitive challenges. Great idea. However, even a clinic that specializes in brain injuries didn't point out the obvious, that with her symptoms and the cognitive challenges she was experiencing, traveling alone from rural Montana to a very busy, new, unknown place to undergo a ton of tests with a bunch of strangers might be overwhelming and a lot to take on and do on her own. Unfortunately, they didn't suggest bringing an advocate or friend, or taking notes or making audio recordings of important meetings and sessions. It's as if the clinic didn't have a clue as to who their patient was—someone who would find any one of those tasks difficult and overwhelming. Unfortunately, it also didn't occur to my friend to take a second set of eyes and ears—an advocate—with her.

This goes back to not knowing what you don't know, again.

NOW, HAND THIS BOOK TO YOUR ADVOCATE TO READ, TOO!

Have a conversation with the person you've chosen as your advocate and bounce ideas off them. Ask them to read this book with you and help you through any parts that feel overwhelming.

Ask For Help: Creating Structure and Support

Asking for help and support may be one of the most important things we do for ourselves, yet, we do it infrequently.

■ ■ ■

N ow that you've got an advocate, the next step is asking for help and creating structure and support. My belief and experience is this:

We need each other!

We need each other to grow and to thrive in all we do. Support is the thing that allows us to make solid, well-thought-out decisions. Support is a critical component as we face challenges in life (planned or emergent), such as injury, illness or surgery and the journey back to optimal health. We need each other and we need support and encouragement. As independent as we may think we are, doing it all ourselves is impossible.

In August 2013, the U.S. Census Bureau published a report stating that 27% of U.S. households were single-person, meaning that approximately 32 million Americans live alone.[2] People who live alone really need support.

CONSCIOUSLY CREATING SUPPORT

Support before surgery can help get you prepared. Support after surgery will allow you to rest, knowing you have help in place and things are being handled.

I recommend building in support for an extended period of time. Even if you begin to feel better quickly, the healing and recovery process can sometimes be one step forward, one step back and continue for weeks or months. Oftentimes, once a cast or other visual reminder of surgery or an injury is removed, we think we are (or should be) better, but the truth is, the body is still healing. Without this visual reminder, those around us may also forget that we are still healing. Healing takes place long after a cast or other visual clue of surgery or an injury is removed. During the recovery period it's better to have too much help in place than too little. It's also easier to send someone home than to feel anxious that something isn't getting done or is falling through the cracks.

Even for the most capable individual, preparing for and recovering from surgery is too much to do alone. Health care crises and undergoing treatment can be overwhelming. Healing can also be painful and tiring. Rather than go at it alone, accept your situation and recognize that you will need help and support.

The key to support is asking for help.

WHO SHOULD I ASK FOR HELP?

- **Spouse or partner**
- **Family**: Parents, siblings, relatives. Children (of all ages) can also be helpful with easy tasks such as bringing you something.
- **Friends**. Remember how good it feels to help a friend? Now is the time to let them feel good helping you!
- **Neighbors**. They are close by and can easily and quickly pop over to help.
- **Co-workers**
- **Team members**
- **Spiritual community**
- **Hire someone**: An advocate, caregiver or assistant.

WHY NOT ASK?

Sometimes we don't ask for help because we don't know what to ask for and sometimes it's because we are afraid to ask. When faced with the need to ask for help I've learned to ask myself, "What's the worst thing that could happen?" The answer is always the same, "nothing," or "they could say 'no'," which is what will happen if I never ask. The great possibility, however, is that I'll get the help I ask for and need when I need it.

PEOPLE WANT TO HELP, BUT OFTEN DON'T KNOW HOW

My experience and observation has been that generally people want to help, but they just don't know how to help or what to do. They need direction; the more specific, the better. Help them help you by giving them suggestions or asking for help with specific tasks.

Put people who offer to help to work bringing meals, assisting with chores, caring for children and pets, running errands, helping to get you organized, or with other needs that arise. Help with even simple things can be huge for a person recovering from surgery. Getting a cup of coffee or glass of water for someone using a walker may seem small, but it is big to them! Kids—even a neighbor's kids—can be really helpful with things such as taking the trash to the curb on trash days, getting the mail and newspaper, mowing the lawn, watering houseplants or walking the dog.

KNOW WHO IS AVAILABLE TO HELP AND WHEN

Some people can only help on weekends while others can help during the week. Create a reference list or calendar with people's availability so you can plan ahead. (Use the calendar on page 185 and the template for organizing people who have offered to help on page 186.)

DON'T MAKE PRESUMPTIONS ABOUT WHO YOU THINK CAN OR WILL HELP

Case in point: I have a friend who underwent major surgery that required she be mostly bedbound for several weeks. As she prepared, she was convinced that her 26-year-old daughter, who was married, with a four-month-old baby and a four-year-old toddler, was too busy to bother. She assumed that her 25-year-old daughter, who was married, but didn't have children, would be more of a go-to girl. However, it turned out not to be the case. Her younger daughter became paralyzed by her fear and anxiety surrounding what her mother was going through and withdrew. It ended up being the older daughter who was present and available to help, in spite of her seemingly full plate.

Lesson: Don't prejudge. Those you think can and will come through for you are sometimes the ones who can't and don't. Those you think are too busy, or you expect the least of, may be the ones who show up the most. Easiest way to know for sure? Ask.

KEEP A TO DO LIST HANDY

Your written ongoing "to do" list will be a particularly handy resource when someone says, "Let me know if you need anything." Now you know how to take them up on their generous offer. Your job is to give assignments and then let go and let the person performing the task figure it out. Small tasks with clear objectives are quick and easy for people to understand and carry out correctly. Being able to complete a task will give your support person great satisfaction. A written list will also help you with distribution, so that no one person gets overburdened with too much.

EXAMPLES:

- "Can you take me to physical therapy Tuesday at 10:00 a.m. for the next four weeks?"
- "I need a dozen eggs, pint of plain whole yogurt and a banana." With a specific list, it's easy for a friend to pick up groceries for you when they're at the store.
- "My room's a mess and I feel stuck. Can you help me organize my closet and dresser?"
- "My porch light is out. Can you get a 100-watt outdoor bulb *and* replace it for me?"
- "Please pick up my prescriptions at [INSERT PHARMACY NAME HERE]." Note: If someone picks up a controlled substance for you (such as an opiate-based pain medication), they will need the physical prescription and will be required to provide a valid ID.

What I know now is I didn't have to do it all alone.
The process could have been easier if I'd been better at asking for help and support.

ONLINE CALENDARS FOR COORDINATING SUPPORT

One way to organize support is by setting up an online calendar that your family and friends have access to. This can help relieve you, the patient, from having to coordinate everything, which can be overwhelming and tire you out when you should be resting. Several excellent websites offer free, private calendars to assist patients with coordinating help and support. These websites are interactive and are also great for posting updates and receiving messages from friends and family. Best of all, they allow people to show support and encouragement by taking action. They can see what, where and when you need help (meals, driving, chores, kids, pets, etc.) and sign up.

I have used CARINGBRIDGE.ORG. It was quick and easy to set up and when I shared the link with people it allowed them to see what was needed and easily jump in. This is an especially helpful tool if you live alone or need long-term support and help.

I have a friend who used CaringBridge when her young daughter was in the hospital for an extended period of time. It allowed her to share progress updates quickly and easily without having to take time away from her daughter to make phone calls. It also allowed her friends and family to stay connected by posting notes of love and encouragement and sharing pictures.

ONLINE RESOURCES FOR FINDING AND HIRING SUPPORT

Following surgery, some people may need additional or long-term help. This may be especially true for people who live alone or who are older and less mobile. Depending on a patient's procedure and progress, some patients are sent home with orders for home health care, which will be arranged by the hospital social worker. However, some patients may benefit from additional support. If that describes you, perhaps hiring some additional part- or full-time support on your own—even for just a stint—would be helpful.

I have used CARE.COM with great success to hire caregivers. What I appreciate about this resource is that CARE.COM is dedicated to the care industry (connecting people in need with caregivers, personal assistants, child care, pet care and housekeeping) and I was able to easily and quickly find qualified candidates. In addition to some excellent candidates, I found it affordable. Basic caregiving in California ranged from $12-15/hour compared to the $20-60/hour I had previously been paying for caregivers hired through agencies.

I know others who have used CARE.COM to find reliable childcare and personal assistants. I also know people who have used CARE.COM to find good jobs.

HOW ELSE DOES SUPPORT LOOK?

Support has many faces. For example, I live in Salt Lake City, Utah and my family lives in Southern California. After my head injury I needed a great deal more support and structure than I had living alone in Utah, so I moved back to California where I first lived with my brother and then a friend. In this case, support looked like living with someone who could provide needed structure and encouragement and assist me with some daily activities, such as going to the market, as I healed.

Years later, when I was able to move back to Salt Lake City, support looked like me living with a friend for six months while I reintegrated back into my Salt Lake life before living independently in my own home. After moving home, knowing I was struggling with some day-to-day basics, such as meal preparation and eating enough, I received support from a kind and generous neighbor who brought me hot meals several times a week. This made such a difference in my level of success. Thank you Jason!

Years earlier, I had reconstructive knee surgery and was wholly unprepared for the magnitude of the healing and recovery process. In that instance, support looked like a friend staying overnight with me after I got home from the hospital and my father getting on a plane and flying out from California and staying with me for close to a month. He did the grocery shopping, cooking and cleaning. He let me beat him at backgammon and ferried me back and forth to physical therapy, all while sleeping on a futon. Thanks, dad! I don't know what I'd have done without you.

For a more recent back surgery I was better prepared. This time I asked my mother *in advance* if she could stay with me for a few days after I got home. She accepted and, in addition, she became a great advocate for me before surgery, too. She went to doctor's appointments with me

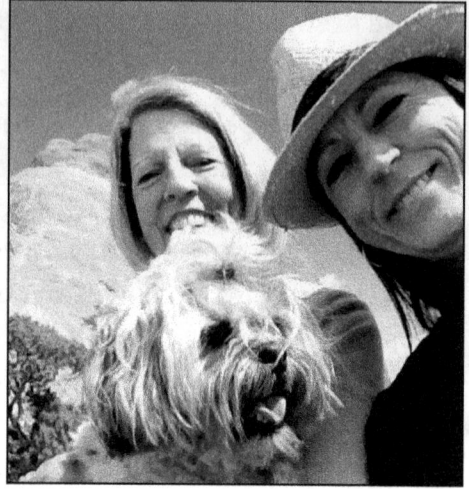
Mom & Bert. Great support team!

and patiently listened when I had the occasional meltdown. How grateful I was after surgery as she checked my incision, helped me with ice, cooked, did errands and laundry, got the mail and cared for Bert so I could rest and heal. Thank you, mom!

I have also had the opportunity to view recovery and support from the vantage point of a caregiver. On one assignment I was hired to provide support to a 65-year-old woman who was recovering from lumbar spinal fusion surgery. Her hospital discharge instructions were to: (1) lie flat on her back with her knees up and rest, so that the fusion process could take place; (2) follow up in the surgeon's office in two weeks to get the surgical staples removed and (3) see the doctor again in six weeks to see how the fusion was progressing. In this caregiving position I lived with her for three weeks. Each day I checked her incision, assisted her in being comfortable, prepared meals, grocery shopped, did errands, managed home health nursing aides (who came to check her vital signs and help her shower), cleaned the house, did laundry, cared for her four cats and took her to follow-up doctor appointments. Going from being a strong, independent woman (she had been a truck driver for over 20 years), to having to lie flat on her back for several weeks was a big challenge for her, so I also provided encouragement and was her sounding board when she needed to talk or vent. Having support and structure in place allowed her to let go of the day-to-day and simply rest and focus on healing.

Questions To Ask Caregivers and Support Team

∎ ∎ ∎

Plan ahead, if possible. Help your family and friends help you by communicating your needs clearly; they aren't mind readers and may assume that if you haven't asked for help, you have everything handled.

Start by creating a list and asking for help

- ☐ Can you help me get organized?
- ☐ Would you be available to watch my children while I am having surgery (or am hospitalized)?
- ☐ Would you stay overnight in the hospital with me?
- ☐ While I am in the hospital can you take care of my pets? Water my plants?
- ☐ Can you bring me something healthy to eat while I'm in the hospital?
- ☐ _____
- ☐ _____
- ☐ _____
- ☐ _____

When I'm home, would you be available if I need help with:

- ☐ Getting in and out of bed (or a chair) and moving around
- ☐ Showering (or bathing)
- ☐ Lifting
- ☐ Moving things around once I'm home and better know what I need
- ☐ Laundry (and putting clothes away)
- ☐ Housework
- ☐ Taking out the trash
- ☐ Getting the mail
- ☐ Watering indoor/outdoor plants
- ☐ Picking up prescriptions

- ☐ Grocery shopping
- ☐ Cooking (and doing the dishes)
- ☐ Childcare
- ☐ Pet care
- ☐ Rides to/from doctor and physical therapy appointments
- ☐ Rides to/from work
- ☐ Errands
- ☐ _____
- ☐ _____
- ☐ _____
- ☐ _____

Creating A Safe and Comfortable Environment

G iven time to plan ahead, a well-organized space can provide structure, support and peace of mind while you are healing.

If you've already had surgery, or it's not possible to do this ahead of time, it's never too late. Getting you organized and creating a safe and comfortable environment are perfect projects for family members or friends wanting to help. The lists on pages 21-32 are filled with ideas. Call a friend and look at the lists together; extra hands and an outside perspective can be invaluable.

ORGANIZING YOUR SPACE—TRY IT ON!

One trick my brother found helpful prior to having surgery was to go into each room and try it on, "as if" he'd already had surgery. For example, knowing he was going to be in bed for a stint, he lay on his bed and imagined how he might be feeling and what he might need or want within arm's reach.

Since he was going to be on crutches for several weeks, he then stood in front of his dresser and imagined being on crutches and how he'd feel. This gave him ideas on how to organize his dresser and clothes for easy dressing. In the bathroom he stood at the sink and again imagined what he'd want within arm's reach. He did the same in the kitchen standing at the stove, the kitchen sink and the refrigerator. Each time he imagined how he might be feeling (standing there on crutches), what he'd want and how he'd manage it. He also sat at the dinner table, at various locations in the living room and on his porch so he could experience what worked and what didn't work. "Trying it on" put him in a headspace that gave him useful information about what would make his post-surgical world easier to navigate.

WHAT MUST GET DONE VS. WHAT WOULD BE NICE TO GET DONE?

If you're feeling overwhelmed by lists and tasks, break them down into things that "must" happen vs. things that would be "nice" to have happen. For example, the dog must be fed and bills must be paid (in theory on time), but getting a haircut before surgery or the car washed might just be nice.

WHAT MUST YOU DO YOURSELF VS. WHAT SOMEONE CAN HELP YOU WITH?

If your "must" list feels overwhelming, break it down further, into things you can do yourself vs. things someone else can help you with or do for you. You have to eat, but someone could (and would probably be happy to) pick up groceries, prepare you something to eat or bring you take-out.

SOME IDEAS TO GET STARTED

Use the ideas on the following pages to help get organized. Spaces are provided at the end of each section to add ideas and items that are unique to your situation that spring to mind. Reminder: Ask for help with these lists.

ORGANIZING YOUR HOME—THE BIG PICTURE

. . .

If you have time before surgery, get as much done as possible. If it's after the fact, have someone help you with these tasks or do them for you. A good rule of thumb is to do whatever will give you peace of mind so that, following surgery, you can rest.

GENERAL HOUSEHOLD ITEMS:

☐ **Organize each room for ease and efficiency**. For example, lie in bed and look around. What can you move now for easier access? Assess each room *"as if"* you've already had surgery. (See example on pages 19-20.)

☐ **If you're going to be on crutches, using a walker or in a wheelchair, do a test run**, if possible. Practice moving around your home using the device to see what might need to be rearranged or moved out of the way. Throw rugs, for example, can be dangerous if you're on crutches or using a walker and should be pulled up for the time being.

☐ **Do you live in a two-story or multiple-level home**? If yes, do you need to temporarily move items onto one level while you're convalescing?

☐ **Set up a comfortable chair outdoors**. If you can, sit outside a little every day. Get some fresh air and soak up some sunshine. Fresh air and sunlight (weather permitting) can be relaxing and contain health benefits. Following surgery, lack of sunshine (coupled with lack of proper sleep) can disrupt natural circadian rhythms, which can trigger depression. Sunshine—bright light—affects brain chemistry, assisting in the regulation of circadian rhythms, which are responsible for producing hormones, chemicals and neurotransmitters. Prolonged sunlight deprivation (being in a dark room or under artificial light for extended periods of time) can cause the wrong amounts of hormones, chemicals and neurotransmitters to be released by the body at the wrong times. This can disrupt the balance and rhythms that govern mood, sleep, appetite and energy. Sunshine can help correct circadian imbalances and aid the path of recovery.

☐ **Laundry**. Coming home from the hospital to clean sheets and clean clothes might feel really nice. If timing doesn't allow for this, ask someone to do it for you. Here's why: Laundry is a multiple-step process that you may not be up to, or capable of doing, for a while following surgery.

☐ **Clean the house**. Does the house really need to be cleaned? If yes, ask for help. Ask someone to do it for you or give yourself the gift of hiring someone to do it.

☐ **Surround yourself with things that make you feel good.** Cozy blankets, soft pillows, favorite pictures. When you are comfortable and relaxed, your body's resources can all be funneled into healing.

THINKING AHEAD—THINGS TO PURCHASE OR TO DO:

☐ **Purchase a bag or two of frozen peas.** Frozen peas make great ice packs, especially for knees, elbows and shoulders; they can be molded to an area and then held in place using an ace bandage. (See pages 48-50 for more on swelling and pages 59-71 for more on pain management, two things ice packs can be useful for.)

☐ **Consider purchasing all-natural wet-wipes.** A wet-wipe bath might feel really good if it's going to be awhile before you are able to tackle a shower or bath. (See pages 42-43 about bathing and showering following surgery.)

☐ **Stock up on movies.** Borrow from a library or sign up for Netflix (NETFLIX.COM), Hulu (HULU.COM), Amazon Prime (AMAZON.COM/PRIME) or other service. My friend has her computer set up so she can stream things from the Internet directly to her television. If you rent movies, be mindful that they will have to be returned on time else late fees could add up. Or, allow for the possibility that following surgery you might just like peace and quiet, to sleep and rest.

☐ **Visit a library or bookstore.** Stock up on books, magazines or puzzles such as Sudoku or crosswords.

☐ **Go to the bank—have some cash on hand.** This is helpful if you need someone to pick something up at the store for you (such as prescriptions or groceries). Cash is also helpful for delivered foods and tipping delivery people.

☐ **Would a handheld showerhead be helpful?** Sitting on a shower chair using a handheld showerhead may be easier and more comfortable after surgery and help conserve valuable energy resources.

☐ **Would installing grab bars be helpful?** Grab bars for balance inside and outside the shower, tub, toilet and bathroom area may be helpful. Depending on your unique situation and needs, grab bars may be helpful in hallways and other areas as well.

☐ **Fill the gas tank in your car.** This is just one less thing to remember or do once you're back on your feet and is courteous if others will run errands with your car.

☐ **Pre-pay regular monthly and re-occurring bills.** Set up online payments or write checks for services such as mortgage or rent, utility and phone bills, health insurance, auto insurance and credit cards. Remembering to pay bills and write checks might be a challenge after surgery; take care of it in advance, if possible.

HELPFUL ITEMS TO HAVE ON HAND:

☐ **Pillbox organizer.** Helpful for taking medications, vitamins and supplements on time. Pillboxes are available at any drug store and come in various sizes. I have one and love it. It alleviates my having to try and remember what to take and when, especially when I've had to take pain medication. Having a neat box also allows me to leave the clutter of pill bottles out of sight, in a drawer.

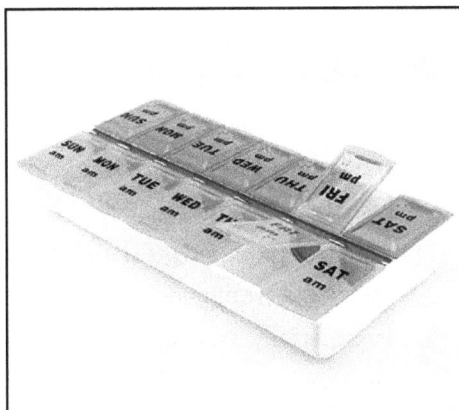

☐ **Do you need a backpack, shoulder bag, pocket belt or basket to carry things?** If you will be on crutches, using a walker or in a wheelchair following surgery, your hands will be full and you may need something to carry items (such as your phone, water bottle, pen, paper, book, etc.) when you move from one room to another. What works for you?

☐ **Would a "long-arm grabber" be helpful?** It can come in handy for reaching or picking things up if you have decreased mobility. Long-arm grabbers are available at hardware stores or via the Internet. For getting dressed, a long-handle shoehorn may be helpful as well. (Note: Depending on your particular insurance, some of these items *may* be covered and given to patients in rehabilitation hospitals.)

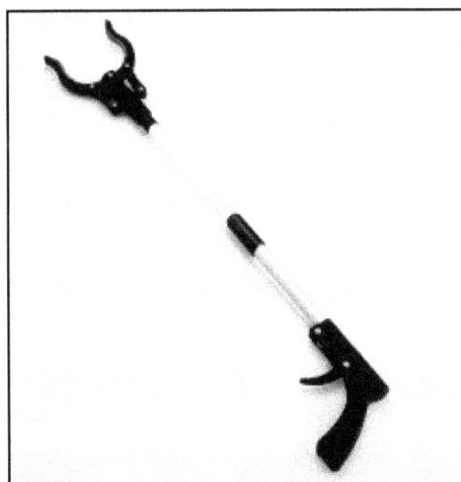

"Long-arm grabber."

SCHEDULING:

☐ **Set your calendar** in advance, if possible. Since doctors and physical therapists can get booked up, set follow-up doctor, physical therapy and other appointments as soon as possible. In doing this you will: (1) avoid any wait to get appointments at busy offices; (2) know your schedule ahead of time and (3) be able to coordinate and arrange for rides. (Keep track of appointments with a monthly calendar. See template on page 185.)

☐ **Make arrangements for the care of loved ones—children and pets.** Whether you're in the hospital or have just come home, would it be helpful if the kids went to grandma's or a friend's for a few days, so you can rest? Do pets need to stay with a friend or can someone come in and take care of them? Cats and goldfish are easy, but dogs need daily care. It might also be necessary to implement some pet management. Dogs and cats that normally jump on the bed can be a problem, startling someone resting or landing on an incision (ouch). Dogs that have a tendency to jump up can also be dangerous because they can cause a patient to lose their balance and possibly fall, especially if a patient is unsteady on their feet.

☐ **Plan for post-surgical driving restrictions**. After surgery, patients are often restricted from driving, sometimes for potentially extended periods of time. This is especially true for patients who have had abdominal, thoracic or right leg surgery. Check with your doctor regarding possible driving restrictions. (See pages 132-133 for more about driving after surgery.)

☐ **Arrange rides to and from the hospital or surgical center**. Following surgery (in- or out-patient), patients are required to have a *reliable* adult drive them home. Driving yourself after any kind of anesthesia or while on pain medication (which can impair your ability to focus, make decisions and react in an emergency) is unsafe and against the law. This is a good job for your advocate or the person you'd like to speak with the doctor and take post-surgical notes on your behalf, before going home.

☐ **If you live alone, arrange to have someone stay with you for *at least* the first 24 hours after you get home**. Since complications and emergencies don't happen on schedule, having someone stay the night once you are home from the hospital or surgical center is essential and for your safety. This is important if you've had out-patient surgery. Today, many procedures that were once performed as in-patient surgeries are now done on an out-patient basis which makes having someone with you even more important. Out-patient surgery can include: orthopedic, back, otolaryngology (ears, nose, throat), gastroenterology (endoscopy), pain manage-ment, podiatry and urology surgeries and procedures, hernia repairs or biopsies, to name a few. Oral surgery, cataract surgery and preventive procedures such as a colonoscopy or elective cosmetic surgery count, too, and require someone be with you for *at least* 24 hours once you are back home.

If possible, have that person stay with you longer than 24 hours. Best-case scenario: Someone is willing to stay with you until your pain is under control and you feel comfortable and confident caring for yourself. This could look like someone staying in your guest room or on your sofa for a night, several nights, a week or longer, depending on the surgery you've had performed and how you are feeling.

If you live alone and it isn't possible for someone to stay longer than 24 hours, arrange to have someone drop by on a regular basis to check in on you and help with tasks. Depending on the surgery and projected recovery it could look like someone stopping by every day or every other day for an hour or two to pick things up off the floor, make you something to eat (and do the dishes), assist with a seated shower, wash your hair, do laundry, move heavy objects, take out the trash, change the cat litter, get the mail, etc. If possible, create a drop-by schedule ahead of time. Having a written list of what you need done can be helpful as well.

ADDITIONAL IDEAS:

☐ _____

☐ _____

☐ _____

☐ _____

☐ _____

PREVENTING FALLS

• • •

Following surgery you may be tired, stiff, sore, weak, dizzy, drowsy or experiencing side effects from pain medication, causing you to be unusually unsteady on your feet and slower to react or respond, putting you at greater risk of a fall.

Anything you can do to keep yourself and your surgical repair safe, such as eliminating obstacles and avoiding falls, is important. Below are some ideas to get you thinking specifically about in-home safety and fall prevention. If you have time before surgery, take a look around your home with these in mind. If time doesn't permit, ask someone to do it for you.

LIGHTING

☐ **Bright lights** in each room will help you see better.

☐ **Make sure there's a light, flashlight or headlamp within easy reach of your bed.**

☐ **Leave a night-light or bathroom light on at bedtime.** Seeing clearly is helpful if you need to get up in the middle of the night.

FURNITURE

☐ **Avoid low or soft furniture.** Some chairs or couches can be difficult to get in or get out of.

☐ **Sit on furniture that has arms.** Dining room chairs, living room chairs and sofas with arms provide leverage and something to lean on as you sit down or get up.

☐ **Stand up slowly after sitting or lying down.** Following surgery, patients can be light-headed. Moving quickly can cause dizziness or blackouts.

CLEAR THE FLOOR

☐ **Clear things from the floor.** Papers, books, clothes, shoes, gym bags, groceries, anything you could possibly stumble or trip over. For those who live with others, especially children, floors must remain clear. Toys, power cords, book bags, etc.

☐ **Temporarily take up throw rugs** or make sure they are securely tacked or taped down.

☐ **Coil or tape cords that run across floors.** Lamp cords and computer cables come to mind.

INDOOR HAZARDS

☐ **Be aware of any medications you're taking that cause dizziness**.

☐ **Lean on a friend, literally.** If you're unsteady, wait until someone is there to lean on or help you move around.

☐ **Wear sturdy shoes.** Comfortable, firm, flat shoes with non-slip soles can provide good support and stability, inside and out. Avoid socks-only or poorly fitted slippers.

☐ **Look for pets before getting up.** Sometimes pets are underfoot and trying to avoid them can cause loss of balance. Pets that have a tendency to jump up can also cause loss of balance.

☐ **Use two hands, even when one will do**. This will help with balance by evenly distributing the weight of any small loads you may be carrying.

☐ **Use the handrail.** If available, use it to support yourself. Following surgery, your balance may be compromised. It's good to be cautious.

☐ **Make sure stairways have secure handrails.** If handrails are there, use them. If not, use extreme caution. Question: Can you or should you be using stairs?

☐ **Check your vision.** Poor vision, or wearing an obsolete prescription, can increase chances of falling.

OUTDOOR HAZARDS

☐ **Make sure hoses are coiled** and other gardening tools and items are out of the way.

☐ **Make note of large cracks in the sidewalk** or uneven pathways.

☐ **Use deicer to melt ice on outdoor walkways in the winter**, if necessary.

OTHER IDEAS OR THINGS TO CHECK:

☐ _____
_____

☐ _____
_____

☐ _____
_____

☐ _____
_____

ORGANIZING YOUR BEDROOM SPACE

■ ■ ■

☐ **Figure out the best way to comfortably and appropriately elevate and support the surgical area.** Do you need to elevate an arm, elbow, a leg or knee? Do you need both knees supported while lying flat, such as after back surgery? Stage pillows and blankets nearby.

☐ **Place clothes you are going to wear (socks, underwear, pajamas, sweats, etc.) in convenient, easy to access places.** Put frequently used items on top of dressers to avoid bending or opening heavy awkward drawers.

☐ **Choose clothing that will fit easily and comfortably over an incision or brace.** Your surgical site may be swollen, bandaged, in a cast or immobilizer, so consider loose-fitting clothes, dresses, button-up shirts or robes. (For example, you're going to need shirts and pajamas that button up the front if you can't raise your arms after shoulder surgery.) Make sure clothing doesn't rub or irritate an incision.

☐ **Choose cotton underwear.** Why? Because cotton is a natural fiber that breathes; it allows the circulation of air. Nylon and other synthetic materials don't, which can cause moisture from perspiration to get trapped, potentially fostering the growth of bacteria and yeast. After surgery you want to eliminate anything that could impede your recovery.

☐ _____

_____

☐ _____

_____

☐ _____

_____

☐ _____

_____

Organizing Your Recovery Area—
What do you need within arm's reach?

. . .

Essentials:

- [ ] **Lamp or light**
- [ ] **Glasses**, if you need them to see or read.
- [ ] **TV remote controls** (with fresh batteries)
- [ ] **Cell phone and charger** (or home phone)
- [ ] **Emergency numbers.** Keep a written list of contact numbers for doctors and the hospital nearby in the event of an emergency. (See template on pages 178-179.)
- [ ] **Medications.** Pillboxes (see example on page 23) can omit some pill bottle clutter on a bedside table and increase your chances of taking medications on time.
- [ ] **Water.** Athletic water bottles or flexi-straws can be an easy way to drink water when lying down. Extra water following surgery is important. (See pages 87-88 for more on the importance of hydration.)

Other ideas:

- [ ] **Alarm clock.** Medication reminders can be helpful if you're drowsy or dozing.
- [ ] **Tissues or handkerchief**
- [ ] **Earplugs.** If you live in a noisy household or neighborhood, earplugs are great for blocking out the world.
- [ ] **Your medical journal.** (See page 118 for ideas on what to include.)
- [ ] **Notepad and pens**
- [ ] **Calendar**
- [ ] **Radio, CD player or iPod.** Stock up on relaxing, healing music or books on tape.
- [ ] **Movies**
- [ ] **Reading materials:** Books, magazines, newspapers, Sudoku, crossword puzzles
- [ ] **Laptop computer and power cord**
- [ ] **"Grabber"** (See image on page 23.)
- [ ] **Pee bucket or bedside commode**
- [ ] _____
- [ ] _____
- [ ] _____
- [ ] _____

ORGANIZING YOUR BATHROOM SPACE

• • •

☐ **Toileting**. After surgery, low toilet seats may be difficult to use. A raised toilet seat with handrails can be a great tool. Installation of a raised toilet seat with handrails does not require permanent changes to your bathroom; it simply sits above your existing toilet.

☐ **Place non-slip carpets on bathroom floors.** Tile, linoleum and hardwood floors can be slippery and dangerous, especially when wet. Wet floors can be even more dangerous if you're on crutches or your balance is impaired from pain or pain medication.

Raised Toilet Seat & Safety Rails

☐ **Evaluate the best way to keep incisions dry when bathing or showering after surgery.** One technique is to cover the area with a plastic bag held in place with tape or rubber bands. Place these items by the shower or tub so you don't have to go looking for them later. (See pages 42-43 for more on bathing and showering following surgery.)

☐ **Would a shower chair (or stool) be helpful?**

☐ **Put a rubber mat in the shower/tub for traction.**

☐ **Place soap, sponge, razor, shampoo and towels within easy reach.**

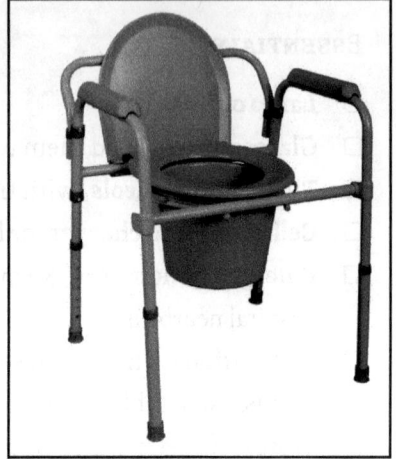

☐ _____
_____

☐ _____
_____

☐ _____
_____

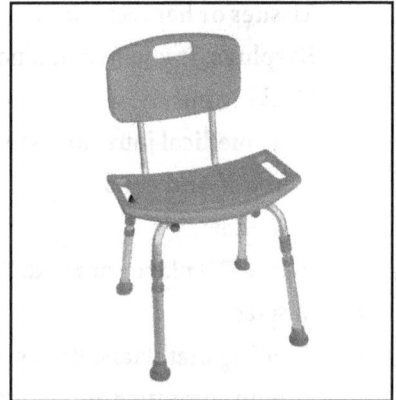

Shower Chair (stool with back)

☐ _____
_____

(See page 133 for ideas and resources for renting items such as a shower chair, raised toilet seat and other helpful assistive devices.)

Organizing Your Kitchen Space and
Prepping Meals and Snacks

■ ■ ■

☐ **Place frequently used kitchen items (especially heavy pots, blender, etc.) on easy to access countertops.** This will help avoid any unadvised lifting, straining or other movements such as bending or twisting.

☐ **Arrange cupboards and drawers so frequently used items are within easy reach.**

☐ **Organize the refrigerator** with commonly used items on easy-to-reach refrigerator shelves.

☐ **Stock up on groceries.** Buy healthy foods that are quick and simple to prepare. Fresh is best. Incorporate extra vegetables and fruits and eliminate highly processed or boxed foods. This will help digestion, assist with keeping blood sugar level and even ease constipation that can accompany surgery. There are many fresh, healthy, prepared food choices available today. For example, some stores have a good variety of pre-made green salads (with or without meat) in the refrigeration section or delicious tuna, tofu and chicken curry salads available in the deli, which are great alone, on crackers or on a bed of lettuce. Some stores also have healthy hot soups, sautés and salad bar options. (See pages 77-86 for more on eating for healing and pages 54-57 for more on the role diet plays in alleviating constipation.)

☐ **Prepare meals ahead of time.** If timing permits, stock the refrigerator and freezer for the first week or two following surgery. Homemade soups, chili and other meals, dished into individual serving containers and frozen, make for simple, easy to heat-and-eat meals. Hard-boiled eggs and quiche made ahead of time are also good protein snacks.

☐ **Ask friends and family to bring in meals.** Let them know your favorite foods and be sure they are aware of any diet restrictions or preferences you may have. A freezer full of turkey soup isn't helpful if you're a vegetarian. Remind them if you have allergies or sensitivities, such as gluten- or dairy-intolerance. Ask them to break meals into single-serving containers.

   A brilliant and inspired idea. My friend Merle had a friend, Jane, who lived alone and fell, badly breaking her leg. Following six weeks in a rehabilitation facility, Jane was faced with months using a walker and an inability to drive. With this in mind, once Jane was home from rehab and feeling able, Merle invited her and several of their mutual friends over for pizza and salad (this included

31

arranging a ride to and from for Jane). In addition to celebrating a safe return home with thanks-giving, each guest was asked to bring a healthy dish for Jane's freezer. Result: An evening that rained love, support and generosity (which I believe positively influences healing) and a freezer full of delicious homemade meals. Thank you Merle!

☐ **Other kitchen and meal ideas** _____

_____

☐ _____

_____

☐ _____

_____

☐ _____

_____

☐ _____

_____

2: UNPLANNED OR EMERGENCY SURGERY

Emergencies—including emergency surgery—occur every day.
What do you need first?
What do you do first?

. . .

Emergencies can be challenging, scary and overwhelming. If this describes the situation you find yourself in, the first thing to know is,

You and the human spirit possess infinite strength—you can do this!

In an emergency situation things may happen at an accelerated pace and you may not have the luxury of making some choices. In fact, there may be a lot of decisions you don't have control over. For example, if you go to the doctor for hip pain and they recommend a hip replacement you may have time to research the surgery, the surgeon, the hospital and the recovery. However, if you fall and break your hip, you will likely need to undergo emergency surgery where you may not have the liberty of choosing your orthopedic surgeon or hospital, or a chance to plan the timing. Depending on the gravity of a situation, it could mean immediate surgery is performed by the surgeon on-call.

IN AN EMERGENCY, WHAT DO I NEED TO KNOW RIGHT NOW?

☐ **Pick up the phone and call someone (a family member, friend or advocate) who can come to the hospital—right now.** (If you can't make the call yourself, give the person's name and number to a nurse and ask them to make the call for you—*right now.*[ii]) Having someone you know and trust by your side during an emergency is crucial. There can be a lot to consider and deal with; too much to undertake alone.

☐ **Bring serious or life-threatening allergies to the attention of doctors and nurses.** If they are life-threatening, stay vigilant.

☐ **Take a deep breath and let go.** Not everything is going to get resolved right now.

■ ■ ■

ONCE YOU ARE STABILIZED AND OUT OF DANGER, THEN WHAT?

☐ **Make sure you understand what's taking place** now and in the immediate days to come.

☐ **Ask for help generating a plan for the future**—for your hospital stay, release, healing and recovery. Include plans for any temporary stay in a rehab facility, the transition home, physical therapy, etc. While doctors, nurses and therapists will be addressing and caring for your physical needs in the hospital, the social work staff at the hospital will be the ones helping with future plans and needs.

☐ **Ask a family member or friend to organize and prepare your home for your return.** Note: If a patient is incapacitated, someone *simply taking the initiative* and doing this for them would be incredibly helpful. (The information and checklists provided on pages 21-32 are a good resource for anyone wanting to help. Ask them to do a walkthrough of your home with your specific needs in mind. Having your home set up prior to your arrival will make for an easier transition.)

[ii] Since much of the population has cell phones these days, we aren't required to memorize important telephone numbers of our family and friends like we did in pre-cell phone times. Having a couple key phone numbers memorized is valuable, especially in an emergency, if you get separated from your cell phone!

SOME FIRST-HAND EXAMPLES DEALING WITH EMERGENCIES

One Saturday afternoon my mom called from an ambulance on the way to the hospital—she'd fallen and was in terrible pain and was understandably scared and anxious. Since I live in Utah and she in California, as soon as we hung up I phoned one of her friends and asked them to meet her at the hospital. Then I phoned my brother who lives nearby to see if he could stay the night at the hospital with her. As my mother's advocate, I knew she needed someone to physically be with her and someone local to advocate for her. I needed someone local to be my eyes and ears, help collect information and see what steps needed to take place next so a plan could be formulated. A couple of days later, after under-going emergency surgery, my mom shared with me that,

> *Knowing she had someone taking care of business—an advocate—made her feel safe.*
> *It allowed her to let go and stop trying to control everything and rest.*

■ ■ ■

During my freshman year at college (I was in Arizona and my family was in California) I was on crutches for a sprained ankle. One day, while balancing crutches and trying to open a heavy steel dormitory door by myself (good reminder about asking for help!), I lost my grip and the door slammed on my good foot. I kept my cool, but knew it was serious. I calmly sat down and had someone call a trusted friend. He picked me up and took me to an emergency room where he held my hand as the doctor examined the injury, stitched it up and cast it up (a partially-severed Achilles tendon). Thank you Jay!

However, now with two injured feet, I was stuck and unable to move around on my own. I was grateful when Jay offered to stay for a couple of days to help me—I

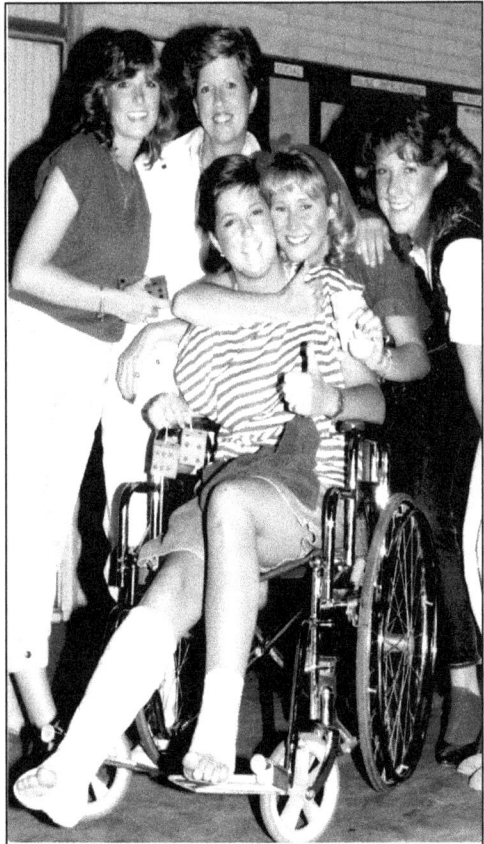

Mom (top center), me (in the wheelchair) and friends, ASU, Tempe, AZ, circa 1985.

didn't know what to do and was also in quite a bit of pain. I was also grateful (and fortunate) my mom was able to come out and help me organize around the injury. Being in a wheelchair for a month and on crutches for an additional four months during school had me experiencing life from a very different perspective and created all kinds of new challenges. It was tricky. I had to learn to ask for help—a lot of help—from friends (and strangers). Turns out help was available, including from my school's disability resource center which provided transportation to and from class. I learned there was a lot to learn and I didn't know what I didn't know. However, in each situation I've encountered I found that asking for help was the first—and most valuable—step. Sometimes it takes a village.

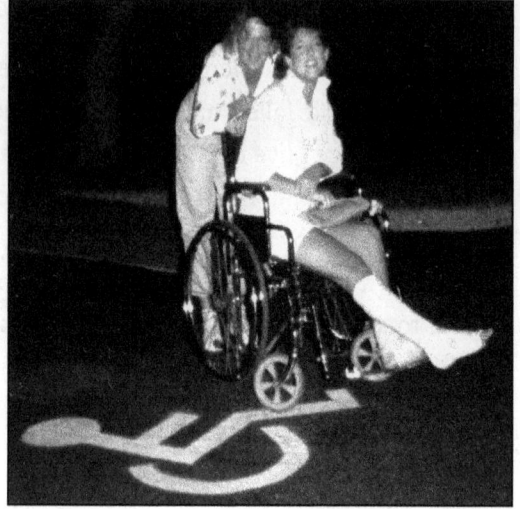

3: BACK HOME—HEALING AND RECOVERY

Healing and recovery are part of the surgical process.
Being mentally and emotionally prepared for this ahead of time will make it easier.

. . .

Back at home after surgery, the important work of healing begins. Since you have just invested the time and expense to undergo a surgical procedure intended to aid your health, allow your body the time and care it needs to heal.

HEALING TAKES TIME

The first thing to know: healing is a process that takes time—quicker for some and slower for others. The only way through it is one day at a time. Depending on the extent of your surgery and its complexities, recovery can be as easy as resting for a couple of days or it can take weeks or months before you feel "back to normal." Each person's recovery and recovery pace are unique; allow for your own experience to unfold.

It's helpful to remember that a "good day," where you are feeling better, can be followed by one, two or even three "bad days" where you just feel crummy. Everyone experiences these ups and downs; they are part of the normal healing process. Know that *you are healing* and that *you will feel better* and get better, even if it feels like one step forward and two backward.

Like many recovering patients, I have experienced this feeling. Resist the urge to judge your progress or compare yourself or your experience to anyone else's, even if they've had a similar procedure. (If you find yourself struggling with the ups and downs and length of recovery right now, jump ahead to pages 102-113 and read about the post-op blues and easing symptoms of the post-op blues and depression.)

BE A PATIENT PATIENT

While general medical guidelines and timelines for healing may exist,

> *Nothing is exact when it comes to recovery or healing;*
> *it simply takes as long as it takes.*
> *Patience is crucial!*

If you've just undergone surgery, even "minor" surgery, be prepared to spend time resting. Often people require more rest than they've anticipated or prepared for. Sometimes healing requires downshifting further than originally planned. Compassion and patience are critical in the recovery phase. "Easy does it" and "one day at a time" are good mantras. It can also be helpful to focus on daily improvements and milestones (even the small ones) rather than focusing on what you cannot do during this time. Become a patient patient.

For example, following my traumatic brain injury, I suffered from debilitating headaches and I slept a tremendous amount. At the beginning, for me a milestone was getting out of bed. Later, walking to the end of the driveway. I remember celebrating the day I realized it had been two days between headaches—that was a huge milestone. Then I celebrated a week between headaches, then two weeks. Happily, those headaches are a thing of the past, but it was years before I hit that milestone. I learned early on in my recovery to be patient and let go. *I couldn't control or think my way to wellness; I had to allow it to occur.*

THINGS MAY TAKE LONGER TO GET DONE

Following surgery you may be moving slower than usual and normally simple tasks may take longer—possibly much longer—than usual. Getting up in the morning, dressing, walking or moving around may be a slower. Preparing something to eat and cleaning up may take longer. Making the bed may feel harder and more laborious, or be impossible for the time being. These are things to accept rather than to judge or get frustrated about. Ask for help and know that it will get better.

I remember recovering from open-heart surgery; in the beginning, simply getting up, getting dressed and having breakfast took until afternoon and in the beginning required a post-breakfast nap. After knee surgery, grocery shopping (on crutches) was a challenge that required extra time, a friend or supermarket clerk to help me and a ride. In these cases I found that instead of muscling my way through a project, accepting that this was how it was going to be for a while made my life and the experiences much easier. Acceptance and patience were my friends.

STRESS-STRAIN DISORDER

As you begin the healing process, in addition to surgical pain and soreness, you may also notice soreness or stiffness, even swelling, in parts of your body not directly associated with the surgery. This may be because you are sleeping, walking, limping, hunching or moving differently than usual due to post-surgical restrictions and pain, or in an effort to protect a surgical site. This is sometimes referred to as stress-strain disorder and it is normal. While it may feel daunting and like "Now what?", try not to focus on or worry too much about it. As you heal and your surgical pain resolves, these other aches and pains will also likely resolve themselves. Hang in there!

VISITORS, THE GOOD NEWS/BAD NEWS

Whether you're in the hospital or back home, consider limiting visitors, especially children. I found visitors to be the good news/bad news. The good news is that it feels good when someone comes to see you. The bad news is that visiting expends a great deal of energy; energy that you may not have, or energy that may be better channeled into healing. Tip: Keep visits short; it's okay to tell visitors you're tired. Thank them for visiting and let them know you need to rest. A good visitor will keep visits brief, or be prepared to just be there with you, content to sit and read or knit or whatever while you sleep and rest.

AT HOME—POST-SURGERY CARE

The following sub-chapters are intended to provide you with knowledge and information for when you are home. They are not a substitute for the medical advice of your doctor. Discuss any concerns or decisions about treatment, care and follow up with your health care provider.

INCISION CARE

. . .

After surgery you will have an incision which may be closed with staples, sutures (also known as stitches), surgical glue (like Krazy Glue), steri-strip elastic skin closures or a combination thereof. The incision may be covered by a bandage or dressing and there may or may not be a tube in or near the incision to allow for fluid drainage.

At the hospital or surgical center your surgeon and nurses will do all your incision care for you. However, at home the responsibility of checking the incision and changing the bandage is yours. To learn how to correctly change your bandage, watch carefully when your surgeon does it. See what your incision looks like underneath the bandage, so you will recognize any differences when you change your bandage at home—whether the wound looks better or worse. It is a good idea to have your advocate or care person available when the doctor demonstrates a bandage change so more than one person knows what needs to be done and how.

Making sure your incision is healthy is important.

REMEMBER, IT'S DELICATE

After surgery, your incision site, while ably held together, is tender and vulnerable. Protect it. The obvious is not to bump or fall on your incision. Protecting it also includes carefully following doctor's post-surgical instructions such as:

- **Appendage use (or non-use)**
- **Movement restrictions** (twisting, bending, lifting, stretching, straining, etc.)
- **Use of a sling or brace, crutches or other assistive device**

There are also less obvious things to consider. For example, if you are experiencing constipation or difficulty urinating, straining to have a bowel movement or to urinate can increase pressure in your system (especially the abdominal area) thereby putting stress on your incision. This kind of straining can be particularly damaging after a surgery such as open-heart surgery. Avoiding and managing constipation following surgery is important. (See pages 51-57 for more on constipation: how to help prevent it and how to help relieve it.)

TIPS TO HELP YOUR INCISION HEAL QUICKLY:

- ☐ **Follow your doctor's instructions**
- ☐ **Wash your hands** before (and after) touching the area
- ☐ **Inspect your incision** daily
- ☐ **Keep the incision area clean and dry**
- ☐ **Protect the surgical area**

CHECKING YOUR INCISION

Keeping an eye on your incision will allow you to quickly recognize any changes.

Check your incision daily, just like your doctor did, to make sure it is not showing any signs of infection, is completely closed[iii] and is healing properly. If your incision is located on your back or an area you cannot clearly see, you will need to ask someone to check it for you. If there is excessive redness, itching or drainage, this may indicate the beginning of an infection, which you will want to catch and treat immediately. (See pages 44-47 for signs and symptoms of an infection or other complication.)

Keep your hands and the incision area clean. Unless specifically recommended by your doctor, resist any temptation to clean your incision with peroxide or alcohol, slather it with first aid ointment (such as Neosporin), or apply powder (in an effort to alleviate itching). These may actually slow the healing process by causing an infection, scarring or other unwanted complication.

Do not pick at scabs. Scabs protect the incision and promote wound healing beneath the surface. Do not remove sutures, staples or steri-strips yourself. Your doctor will do this for you, when the time is right. Removing sutures too early, or incorrectly, may cause the incision to reopen and again, may result in infection, scarring or other complication.

KEEP YOUR INCISION(S) DRY

It is usually recommended that you keep an incision dry until it's completely healed and any scab has fallen off. This is because: (1) bath, shower or pool water (including ocean, lake or river water) is not sterile and can introduce infection into an incision and (2) exposure to water can cause an incision to soften and open. (See page 42 for ideas on how to keep an incision site (or sites) dry.)

[iii] A wound that opens is a condition called dehiscence, which should be reported to your doctor.

BATHING AND SHOWERING

. . .

Bathing and showering are important aspects of incision care. Proper cleanliness can help ward off infection. Instructions for safe bathing and showering should be provided when you are discharged from the hospital or surgical center. If not, ask. The location of your surgical site will help determine whether a bath or shower is more advisable. Additionally, while a hot shower or bath might sound good following surgery, it may not be the best thing for you. Sitting in a hot tub or standing in a hot shower both expend a great deal of energy and can place undue stress on the body's systems which can be fragile following surgery.

When you embark on your first bath or shower, having someone nearby is a wise safety precaution. No one ever plans on slipping or falling, but surgical patients are a greater fall risk due to instability, light-headedness, fatigue, pain and side effects from some medications. If you are alone, err on the side of caution and wait for someone to come home or come over prior to bathing or showering. If you're unstable or uncomfortable in any way, ask someone to assist you.

WET-WIPE OR SPONGE BATH

Before tackling a bath or shower following surgery, it may be easier to start simple, such as with a wet-wipe or sponge bath and work up from there. A wet-wipe or sponge bath is a great way to freshen up following surgery if you're not quite ready for a bath or shower. You can do it yourself in bed or ask someone help you.

Note: Most commercial wet-wipe products available in supermarkets and drug stores are filled with chemicals and artificial ingredients, including strong perfumes which can be especially overwhelming to the senses after surgery. Try natural, hypoallergenic herbal wipes, which have anti-microbial properties and are free of artificial fragrances, dyes, parabens (chemical preservatives) and phthalates.[iv]

BATHING

If your incision is located on an appendage or area of the body that can be easily kept above the water's surface, bathing would be recommended. Don't bathe if the incision

---

[iv] Phthalates are chemical plasticizers added to products to increase their flexibility, transparency, durability and longevity. Since manufacturers aren't required to list phthalates separately, it can be challenging to tell which products contain them. Many products include phthalates under the term "fragrance."

would be submerged in bath water, making it vulnerable to bacteria in the water or to softening and opening.

If the possibility exists that your incision could get wet while you are in the tub, take precautions and protect it with a waterproof bandage or plastic bag secured by a rubber band or tape.

SHOWERING

Depending on the location of your incision, showering may be easier and quicker. Similar precautions should be exercised when showering, most importantly, keeping the incision site dry. If you have a handheld showerhead, use it; it's a great way to control the direction and flow of water away from an incision.

A reminder: Following surgery, standing, even for a short shower, expends a great deal more energy than sitting and might be difficult, painful or dangerous if you are unsteady on your feet. To conserve energy, consider sitting on a chair in the shower. (See examples on pages 30 and 133.) For stability, place the chair on a rubber mat.

SWIMMING

Swimming is contraindicated until an incision is completely closed and any scab has fallen off. Public pools can be a breeding ground for bacteria and germs. Prolonged submersion in pool water can cause an incision to soften and open, leaving it vulnerable and interfering with the healing process.

SIGNS AND SYMPTOMS OF INFECTION

When in doubt, always choose the cautious route and call your doctor.
Early intervention can help prevent serious complications.

■ ■ ■

WHEN TO SEEK EMERGENCY MEDICAL TREATMENT

While the indicators of infection can be frightening to read about, they are simply things to be aware of and are outlined here for your information. Being aware of the signs and symptoms of an infection or other complication is valuable so you can recognize if or when your recovery has changed from "normal" to one that may need medical attention.

Some signs of infection are obvious, such as pus coming out of an incision, while others may be less obvious, such as feeling tired or the appearance of a tiny gap in your incision. If in doubt, call your doctor or surgeon and ask. Ignored, small things can quickly develop into potentially major surgical complications. Better safe than sorry.

There are times when no matter how diligently you care for your incision,
an infection or other complication may still arise.
All you can do is your best.

CALL YOUR SURGEON IF YOU NOTICE OR EXPERIENCE ANY OF THE FOLLOWING:

- **Increased redness at the incision site**. Some redness is normal, but should decrease in both size and redness over time rather than increase in size or get redder.
- **Red streaks (or a rash) on the skin that radiate from the incision site to surrounding areas**.
- **Increased swelling or hardening of the incision**. An infected incision may appear puffy, swollen or gradually harden as the tissue underneath becomes inflamed.
- **Numbness around the incision that spreads or gets worse**.
- **Bleeding or pus coming directly from (or around) the incision**. A small amount of clear drainage from an incision is normal. However, blood, anything that looks cloudy (such as pus) or has a bad odor is a sign of infection. Pus can range in color from blood-tinged to green, white or yellow and may be thick or chunky.

- **Your incision is hot**. An infected incision may feel hot to the touch, which is caused by the body sending infection-fighting blood cells to the area.

- **A fever over 101°F (38.3°C)**. A low-grade fever of 100°F or less can be normal after surgery, but a fever over 101° may indicate the presence of an infection and should be reported. A fever may cause you to feel chilled, decrease your appetite, lead to dehydration or cause a headache.

- **Pain medicine does not control your pain**.

- **Malaise**. Feeling tired, "blah," "off," lacking in energy or sleeping more than usual may be symptoms of an infection that is moving through your system. These feelings are also common for patients who are recovering from surgery who do not have an infection. The difference is that when recovering from surgery you should feel a little better every day, rather than feeling better for a few days then suddenly feeling exhausted and lethargic for no apparent reason.

Signs of Other Potential Surgical Complications

. . .

Again, following surgery you should be feeling a little better each day. If any of the following occur they may indicate a complication and should be reported to your doctor.

PAY ATTENTION TO:

- **An incision that opens or begins to pull apart.** If your incision begins to separate, cover the wound with a clean bandage to control any drainage and contact your surgeon. Sometimes, this complication can be prevented by holding or applying a little pressure on an incision when sneezing, coughing or rising from a chair.
- **Sudden onset of severe, unexplained, uncontrollable pain.** Following surgery your pain should slowly steadily diminish as you heal. (A slight increase in pain can be normal if you overdo it with an activity or you decrease your pain medication.)
- **Unexplained leg pain.** One risk of surgery, or inactivity due to surgery, is the development of blood clots in the legs, known as deep vein thrombosis (DVT), which can be caused by durations of little to no body movement. (This is one reason it's good to get moving and keep moving following surgery.) Blood clots can be dangerous as they can travel through the bloodstream to the lungs or brain causing difficulty breathing, a stroke or other complication.[3] Unexplained leg pain may be an indicator of DVT.
- **Difficulty breathing.** Pay attention to any changes or problems with your breathing following surgery. A change in your ability to breathe is significant and may indicate a serious problem, such as a blood clot in the lung.
- **Coughing or vomiting blood.** This can indicate blood in the stomach or lungs and can be a potential medical emergency. Note: Blood from the stomach may not look like blood, but like coffee grounds.
- **Bloody bowel movements.** Unless your surgeon says you might experience blood in your stool for few days after surgery, blood in your stool should be reported.
- **Persistent diarrhea.**
- **Persistent nausea or vomiting.**
- **Not able to eat.** If your surgeon has sent you home from the hospital to recover, you are expected to be able to eat and drink on your own to obtain adequate nutrition to heal. If your ability to eat or drink suddenly changes or you cannot keep food and fluids down, this could indicate a complication of some kind.

- **Increasing weakness or inability to care for yourself.** If you start to feel like you are getting weaker rather than stronger or you're not able to care for yourself, something may be wrong. A decrease in your ability to function, such as not being able to walk to the bathroom, can be a sign of some complication.
- **The worst headache ever.** If you don't usually suffer from headaches and your doctor hasn't told you to expect a severe headache after surgery, the onset of a sudden, severe headache may indicate something serious; tell your surgeon.

Swelling and Inflammation

. . .

In its most basic form, swelling is simply excessive fluid in a given area. Swelling is often a sign of inflammation. Inflammation is the body's reaction to trauma, a foreign body, bacteria, virus or a metabolic imbalance. While not all swelling involves inflammation, most inflammation involves swelling. Additional symptoms of inflammation may include redness, heat and pain.

Surgery is considered a trauma to the body and swelling is a normal part of the healing process; it is the body's first response to any trauma. No matter how well a surgery is performed, any degree of trauma will result in swelling. The amount of swelling following surgery (or an injury) depends on a host of factors including the extent of the trauma and the state of health of the individual prior to surgery.

Following trauma, to protect itself, the body immediately sends coagulators (blood clotting mechanisms) to the traumatized site and the immune system kicks in. The body also automatically sends cells called dendrites and macrophages which clear away debris and damaged cells by literally digesting them. This whole process causes vasodilation, or opening of the blood vessels, which is experienced as swelling.

While some swelling is beneficial (to clean the area and assist healing), too much swelling can interfere with circulation, cause pain and limit range of motion. Excessive swelling may also lead to other complications such as opening an incision.

If you take away all the swelling, you potentially lose some regeneration and healing. Allow too much swelling and you may leave the body vulnerable. What to do? Because of all these factors, doctors are very mindful of inflammation.

FOLLOW YOUR DOCTOR'S INSTRUCTIONS AND USE COMMON SENSE

Different procedures or surgeries will have different post-op recommendations for swelling and inflammation. For example, while ibuprofen is often recommended for alleviating swelling, it is not recommended following certain surgeries; every procedure will have its own specific regimen. The following are guidelines, but check with your doctor.

ICE

Ice is a good tool to reduce swelling (and assist with pain management). Ice is a vasoconstrictor, meaning it causes blood vessels to narrow, limiting internal bleeding at an incision or injury site. Depending on the procedure or injury, ice is traditionally recommended in 20-minute increments (20 minutes an hour on ice for the first 72 hours and then as directed thereafter). This 20-minute rule is important. The notion that if a little ice is good, a lot of ice is better, does not apply. In fact, too much ice (more than 20 minutes an hour) can cause more damage than good, including frostbite. To help prevent frostbite, place a towel or layer of protection between your skin and the ice pack or ice source and set an alarm as a reminder in case you forget or fall asleep. Note: There are some instances where ice is not recommended. Ask your doctor about icing and follow instructions.

Is one ice pack better than another?

Ice pack technology has grown in leaps and bounds and there are now many options on the market, including motorized cold therapy units (as seen on page 134) and ice packs specifically designed to wrap around and mold to shoulders, necks, elbows, wrists, ankles, knees, etc. An online search of "ice packs for shoulders" will net a whole lot of options. A bag of frozen peas also makes a great ice pack as they can be molded to an area and then held in place using an ace bandage. (Note: Refreeze peas before they turn to mush.) Ask your doctor or physical therapist for their recommendations.

What about heat?

Generally, the post-surgical use of heating pads or heat treatments is not recommend-ed. Heat increases circulation, bringing blood into an area. Increased blood flow can cause unwanted swelling, which can cause an increase in pressure and pain.

ANTI-INFLAMMATORIES

Anti-inflammatories, non-steroidal anti-inflammatory drugs (also collectively known as "NSAIDs") and steroids such as cortisol, can be helpful in reducing swelling and are also a type of pain reliever. Most people recognize NSAIDs by their generic names ibuprofen or aspirin and their brand names Advil, Motrin, Midol, Aleve, Nuprin, Bayer or Ecotrin. NSAIDs are fundamentally the same, but one may be more appropriate for a patient, or a patient may respond better to one over another. For instance, in low doses (200-400 mg every eight hours) ibuprofen blocks pain; at higher doses (600-800 mg every eight hours) ibuprofen is also an anti-inflammatory. Taking ibuprofen regularly in the appropriate dose is necessary for efficacy.

It is important to make a distinction between NSAIDs, such as ibuprofen, and other pain relievers such as acetaminophen (also known as Tylenol), because acetaminophen is also frequently prescribed by doctors, but does not control inflammation. Acetaminophen is strictly used for pain and fever reduction.

With most injuries or trauma, such as from surgery, pain is accompanied by swelling. Pain may even be worse because of swelling. While pain and swelling are indicators that ibuprofen may be appropriate, there may be medical or case-specific reasons a doctor prescribes a particular remedy. It's worth asking to be sure.

EAT RIGHT

A healthy diet will provide the body with the essential vitamins and nutrients it needs to heal and repair itself. (See pages 77-86 for more on eating to support healing and recovery.) Some foods, like leafy greens, contain nutritional components that are also helpful in reducing swelling.[v] Pineapple, papaya and turmeric are additionally known for their anti-inflammatory properties.

HYDRATE

Proper hydration (drinking plenty of water) may also naturally help reduce swelling. How? Given that the body is more than 60% water, being properly hydrated allows the body's systems to function optimally, including flushing excess fluids and toxins from surgery. (See pages 87-88 for more on the importance of hydration.)

---

[v] Note: Patients who are placed on blood thinning medications such as Coumadin or Warfarin are often advised to avoid foods containing vitamin K. However, many of the foods that contain vitamin K, such as kale, spinach, collards, greens and broccoli are also rich with other vitamins and minerals that are excellent for health and healing. If you want to include these vitamin-rich healing foods in your diet, tell your doctor and ask them to adjust your blood thinning medication accordingly.

CONSTIPATION

The first and most important thing to know about constipation is
you absolutely want to avoid it!

■ ■ ■

Constipation is defined as the difficulty (or the inability) to pass feces because they are dry, hardened or the bowel's motility is impaired.

Constipation occurs when the contractions of the colon (which is part of the large intestine) are too slow, causing too much water to be drawn out of the stool. As the length of time between bowel movements increases, more water is absorbed out of the colon, back into the bloodstream, causing the stool to further harden in the colon. Constipation becomes more severe the longer it lasts.

Unfortunately, post-surgery patients are far more likely to have
a bout of constipation than the average person.[4]

Many people have shared with me that no one prepared them with information on constipation, especially the fact that pain medication almost always causes constipation.

CONSTIPATION AFTER SURGERY? WHY WORRY?

Constipation is a problem because it stops the body's natural process of elimination which can increase pain levels and place undue stress on the body, including a new incision. Regular elimination is important following surgery so the body can flush toxins from the system and begin to heal.

PREVENTION IS THE BEST MEDICINE!

With regard to surgery-related constipation, it is much easier to care for the bowels before constipation sets in than to get through it once it becomes a problem. If you are naturally prone to constipation, share this detail with your doctor, as you may be at even greater risk following surgery.

PAY ATTENTION

If left untreated, constipation can progress to impaction, which is when the stool is so hard and dry that you cannot have a bowel movement. The hardened stool may then need to be removed using enemas, digital disimpaction or, in advanced cases, surgery. Not fun.

Another reason to avoid constipation following surgery is that straining to force a bowel movement when constipated can cause complications including unusual heart rhythms, hemorrhoids or shortness of breath and can place undue stress on tender new incisions (internally and externally), possibly causing an incision to open.

Patients who have had open-heart and gastrointestinal surgery can be at particular risk from constipation. When the heart is recovering from surgery it cannot tolerate the changes in heart rhythm that straining—bearing down to have a bowel movement—can cause. For patients who have had surgery in the gastrointestinal tract, such as colon surgery or weight loss surgery, constipation can cause damage to the surgical area.[5]

WHY AM I SO CONSTIPATED?

There are many reasons patients are more likely than usual to be constipated following surgery:

- **Anesthesia**. Anesthesia puts the whole body to sleep, paralyzing the intestine along with the rest of your body. This includes halting the contractions that push food through the intestinal tract. Until your intestines "wake up" nothing there moves, including any feces that may be in the intestinal tract. Waking up the intestines can take time, which may cause constipation.
- **Pain medication**. Prescription medication given for pain relief can be very drying to the body and can cause or worsen constipation. If you must take large or multiple doses of pain medication or take pain medication for an extended period of time, you will be at risk.
- **Inactivity**. Spending more time in bed or an easy chair resting after surgery may also trigger constipation. While resting is important, getting up and walking is valuable, too. Activity is one of the body's natural triggers for a bowel movement.
- **Lack of food and water in the body**. As part of your preparation for surgery, you were likely instructed not to eat or drink the night before surgery and after surgery, you may have a restricted diet, be nauseous or not hungry. The combination of little to no food or liquid intake can work against the body's normal routine of elimination, again contributing to constipation. Food and the act of eating stimulate the digestive system and keep things moving. With no food being eaten, the "food in, food out" mechanism doesn't work. Too little fluid in the body also means less fluid in feces which can result in hard dry stools.
- **Diet**. Along with possibly eating or drinking less, your diet may have changed after surgery. For example, if you are hospitalized, the food provided in the

hospital may be a dramatic departure from your normal diet and this can contribute to or worsen constipation.

Following surgery it is important to make good food and beverage choices that support the body's elimination process. While some foods can help prevent, treat and ease constipation, other foods can contribute to or worsen constipation. (See page 56 for some foods that can ease constipation and page 85 for foods and ingredients likely to worse constipation.)

THINGS YOUR DOCTOR CAN DO

Prior to surgery, your doctor may prescribe a medication or recommend an over-the-counter remedy or treatment for constipation, such as a laxative or enema, as a preventive measure. Do not use over-the-counter treatments without first discussing them with your doctor. If you are taking any preventive measures (prescription or over-the-counter, including natural or herbal remedies), tell your doctor what you are taking and the symptoms you are trying to alleviate.

Various remedies for constipation are collectively known as laxatives, available in both over-the-counter or prescription form.

THERE ARE THREE TYPES OF LAXATIVES—EACH WORK A LITTLE DIFFERENTLY

1. **Some soften the stool**, such as Colace, which works by increasing the amount of water the stool absorbs, making the stool softer and easier to pass.
2. **Some act as a bulk agent**, such as Metamucil, which increases bulk in the stool and absorbs water, forming a softer, bulky stool, which can be easier to pass.
3. **Some stimulate the colon**, such as Senna, which stimulates the nerve endings in the walls of the colon, causing contractions (known as peristalsis), moving matter through the intestines and bowel.

Different people, different bodies and different situations may respond better to one treatment versus another.

THINGS YOU CAN DO

Changing how you eat and drink has been documented to positively impact the gastrointestinal (or GI) system. A healthy diet may help prevent constipation from occurring or help ease symptoms if it does develop.

Preparing your bowels prior to surgery and caring for them following surgery can be similar processes. It is important to: (1) eat foods that have the potential to ease symptoms and support elimination such as fresh vegetables, fresh fruits and healthy fats and (2) to drink plenty of water and clear fluids. The bonus is that fresh vegetables, fresh fruits, healthy fats and water are also good for healing.

CONSTIPATION-EASING SUGGESTIONS:

Note: The order in which this list appears is intentional and important.

(1) **HYDRATE**—DRINK WATER

Without water, nothing works properly. Increase water and healthy clear fluids. Increasing your intake of clear fluids such as water, herbal teas and clear broths will help keep you hydrated and can decrease the risk or severity of constipation. Fluids will also help your body recover if you develop constipation. However, Mountain Dew, for example, with its array of chemical additives, does not count as a healthy clear fluid. Avoid highly sugary beverages, such as soda and juice, which can have a drying effect. Sixty-four ounces (or eight 8-ounce glasses) of water a day is recommended. Eight ounces is small, less than a can of soda or a mug of coffee.[vi]

(2) **LUBRICATE**—EAT HEALTHY FATS

All cells require fatty acids and cholesterol to function optimally. An adequate intake of healthy fats is necessary to many functions in the body, including elimination. Healthy fats (which you can get from avocados, coconuts, coconut oil, coconut milk, eggs, olives, extra-virgin olive oil, raw nuts, raw seeds and cold-water fish) are necessary for the absorption of fat-soluble vitamin A, which is critical to building and maintaining the mucosal lining of the colon. Healthy fats can also act as stool softeners, to a degree. Conversely, the lack of healthy fats in the colon can disrupt the peristaltic wave in the colon, interrupting or halting elimination.

(3) **ENCOURAGE PERISTALSIS** (VIA ADEQUATE MAGNESIUM)

Magnesium helps relax the muscles lining the walls of the colon, resulting in smoother, rhythmic contractions which move stools through the colon. It also attracts water into the colon, making for softer stools and has an overall calming effect on the body.

[vi] For some, a morning cup of coffee can initiate a bowel movement, but an excess through the day, can be dehydrating (and negatively impact sleep).

Magnesium can be taken orally by tablet, or by adding a product such as Calm (by Natural Vitality) or Epsom salt (also known as magnesium sulfate, a naturally occurring mineral substance distilled from seawater[vii]) to water.

The average adult can safely take 400 milligrams of magnesium a day to stimulate a bowel movement and can increase by 200 milligrams a day up to bowel tolerance. Taking too much magnesium can cause loose stools or diarrhea and for some, gas or bloating.

While there are no major side effects to taking Epsom salts, more than two doses within 24 hours may cause abdominal pain, diarrhea, bloating or nausea. You may also notice feeling unusually thirsty after taking Epsom salts since they cause a large amount of water to be drawn into the colon. Discuss any questions with your doctor.

(4) INCREASE FIBER

Fiber is the part of plant material we cannot digest that adds bulk and softness to a stool, in turn encouraging a bowel movement. Understanding what fiber does, and which foods are good sources of fiber, can help you make good food choices that will keep your system moving.

Increasing fiber before becoming constipated is a good preventive measure. However, if you are already constipated, wait to increase fiber until after you've had a successful bowel movement.[viii] If your bowels are already dry and you are constipated, avoid consuming a lot of fiber on top, as you won't have the necessary components in place to move feces through the colon. Instead, focus on hydrating, lubricating and encouraging peristalsis (items 1-3) until you have a bowel movement, then increase fiber to help stay regular.[ix]

Once your have had a successful bowel movement, increasing natural fiber is helpful because it serves to both add softness and bulk to a stool. There are two kinds of fiber: soluble and insoluble. Soluble fiber absorbs water and binds with fatty acids, forming a gel-like substance that keeps stools soft. Insoluble fiber does not dissolve in water; instead, it adds bulk to the stool.

[vii] Epsom salt is also great in a bath and is said to ease nervous system tension, relax sore muscles and relieve bruises, swelling and cramps. It can be found in the first aid aisle of any grocery store. I personally love a good soak in Epsom salts and experience it to be soothing, relaxing and healing.

[viii] While too little fiber can cause constipation, adequate fiber can ease constipation and return the bowel and elimination system to normal. Fiber can also be used to help normalize diarrhea; it can be helpful for both.

[ix] For some, too much fiber may cause bloating or diarrhea.

The best foods for constipation are those that contain more fiber. Contrary to popular opinion and what some advertisers would have you believe, wheat products and whole grain foods are not good sources of fiber for everyone.[x] For many, grains can be more problematic than helpful; they can irritate the bowels and cause gas and bloating. Reducing or eliminating "fiber-rich" grains and adding fiber-rich vegetables tends to benefit the most people. Fiber is good, provided it comes from the right source. For example, adding fiber to highly processed, packaged foods containing sugar and artificial ingredients does not make a bad food better. Obtaining fiber through fresh natural foods is best.

Since both soluble and insoluble fiber are found in all plant foods, simply focusing on eating a wide variety of fresh (raw or steamed) vegetables, fruits and legumes may help decrease the risk or severity of constipation and assist the body in returning to its normal elimination schedule.

GOOD SOURCES OF SOLUBLE AND INSOLUBLE FIBER				
VEGETABLES		**FRUITS**		**LEGUMES**
Artichoke hearts	Chard	Apples	Pears	Garbanzo
Asparagus	Green beans	Apricots	Pineapple	Kidney
Brussels sprouts	Kale	Figs		Navy
Broccoli	Peas	Melon		Pinto
Cabbage	Spinach	Papaya		
Carrots	Squash	Peaches		

If increasing fiber-rich foods doesn't solve the problem, you can try adding a fiber supplement. If you are going to use a fiber supplement, check with your doctor and choose a *natural* fiber supplement. Not all fiber supplements are created equal. For example, many people are familiar with brand names, such as Metamucil, but are not aware that in addition to fiber, many of these products also include sugar, aspartame, artificial color and artificial flavor, which are best avoided.

(5) HERBAL LAXATIVES

Use laxatives as a last resort. A natural herbal laxative will generally contain healthier ingredients and may be easier on a delicate post-surgical elimination

---

[x] Wheat, whole wheat and whole grain products such as bread, cereal, rice (including brown rice varieties), crackers, popcorn, pretzels, pancakes, tortillas, etc., are generally poor sources of fiber.

system. Most drug store products contain chemical and artificial additives, which can be taxing to the body. Read ingredients and ask questions to be sure.

OTHER SUGGESTIONS TO PROMOTE A BOWEL MOVEMENT:

- **Eat a significant meal in the morning**. For most people, the system that triggers the urge to defecate is at its peak in the morning. To take advantage of your body's innate knowledge and re-establish a natural rhythm for bowel movements, eat a substantial breakfast to stimulate the gastrocolic reflex. The gastrocolic reflex is caused by expansion of the stomach, which causes the emptying of the colon. Eating triggers intestinal contractions, which move matter through the intestines, resulting in a bowel movement. Note: This does not mean drinking a cup of coffee and eating half a dozen donuts. *What* you eat is as important as *when* you eat.

- **Give it time**. During your recovery, allow time each morning for a relaxing trip to the bathroom following breakfast. Allow your body time to get back into its regular biorhythm. Never force or strain to have a bowel movement.

- **Eat meals regularly throughout the day**. Since the act of eating can stimulate intestinal contractions, it is a good idea to eat something every few hours. Eating meals on a regular and consistent basis can help encourage your system to keep moving. Food in = waste out.

Blood Pressure

. . .

Blood pressure is the pressure exerted by circulating blood upon the walls of blood vessels. High blood pressure (also known as hypertension) requires the heart to work harder than normal to pump and circulate blood. Low blood pressure (also known as hypotension) is the opposite and can deprive the brain and body of an adequate blood supply leading to dizziness, light-headedness or other symptoms.

BLOOD PRESSURE AND SURGERY

If you have high (140/90, or higher) or low (under 90/60) blood pressure, inform your surgeon so it can be properly monitored before, during and after surgery.

If you traditionally have normal blood pressure,
it's reasonable to assume this will continue to be the case.

However, having surgery is stressful on the body and may cause blood pressure to become elevated or depressed. In most cases this is temporary. As your body rests and heals, your blood pressure likely will return to normal as well. Not everyone's blood pressure goes up or down under circumstances such as surgery but, if it does, your doctor may keep you until your blood pressure is back within acceptable limits.

REASONS YOUR BLOOD PRESSURE MAY CHANGE FOLLOWING SURGERY:

- Increased pain
- Anxiety or stress
- New medications
- Shock
- Blood loss/bleeding
- Severe infection
- Severe allergic reaction
- Dehydration

High blood pressure can be especially dangerous with potential serious short- and long-term ramifications including: damaging arteries, stroke (high blood pressure is the leading cause of strokes), aneurysm, heart attack or heart failure.

CONTROLLING YOUR BLOOD PRESSURE CAN REDUCE THESE RISKS

It is easiest to try and control blood pressure through proper diet, nutrition, rest, self-care and exercise, when appropriate. However, if your blood pressure remains abnormally high or low, your doctor may prescribe medication to bring it within normal levels.

PAIN MANAGEMENT

Pain is the body's way of communicating directly with you.
"Please pay attention. Stop what you're doing. Wrong way."

∎ ∎ ∎

Pain control and pain management are important aspects of your post-operative care and recovery. Pain is our body's natural response—indicator—that something isn't right or we are doing something it doesn't like. It is there to stop us from continuing an activity that may be harmful.

Pain also occurs to slow us down so we can heal. Excessive unrelenting pain, however, can hinder and impede recovery by interfering with the body's ability to relax and rest. Proper pain management facilitates recovery, improves a patient's quality of life and can prevent additional health complications.

THERE ARE TWO PRIMARY CATEGORIES OF PAIN:

(1) **Acute pain**, which is pain that takes place after surgery (or an injury), before healing has occurred. Acute pain generally resolves and disappears as the underlying cause of the pain resolves and heals. Following surgery, most patients experience some acute pain that should subside a little each day.

(2) **Chronic pain**, which is long-term pain that generally lasts more than six months.

THE GOAL OF POST-SURGICAL PAIN MANAGEMENT IS TO REDUCE PAIN SO HEALING CAN TAKE PLACE

While you are in the hospital, communicate with your doctors and nurses about your pain level so appropriate measures can be taken to alleviate unnecessary suffering. Tell them about pain medications that have worked well (or not so well) for you in the past. Include any history of adverse reactions to—or prior abuse issues with—any controlled substance so your medical team can devise the best possible pain management plan specifically for you.

Generally, with respect to pain management following surgery, it is advisable to stay ahead of the pain—manage the pain along the way—rather than waiting for pain to become unbearable and then seek intervention.

It's easier to manage and prevent pain
than to try and chase significant pain after the fact.

THE BENEFITS OF PAIN CONTROL AND PAIN MANAGEMENT INCLUDE:

- **The ability to be discharged sooner from the hospital.**
- **Greater comfort as you heal.** When pain is under control, it allows you to relax so healing can take place.
- **The ability to sleep**, relax and rest, which are paramount in healing.
- **Decreased stress and anxiety caused by severe pain.**
- **Gaining strength back more quickly.** Less pain allows a patient to move more easily, breathe more deeply and walk sooner which promote healing. Post-surgical activity may also reduce the risk of developing certain complications such as pneumonia, blood clots, pulmonary and cardiac complications, the development of neuropathic (or chronic) pain and constipation.
- **Stabilizing blood pressure, heart rate, appetite and general mood.** These, and other body systems, can all be negatively affected by excessive or uncontrolled pain.

HEALING OCCURS FASTER WHEN PAIN IS UNDER CONTROL

Less pain will advance your recovery and aid you in returning to full function sooner. However, rather than expecting your recovery to be pain-free, pay attention to what increases your pain. Be cautious and let pain be your guide.

If pain gets significantly worse following an activity, that's your indicator you've done too much or you've done something your body may not be ready for. If pain continues to significantly increase, it may indicate the presence of something else going on. This is the time to call your doctor to assess and determine whether what you are experiencing is "normal" or if you need to be seen in the office.

NOTE TO CAREGIVERS, FAMILY MEMBERS AND FRIENDS:

When someone is in significant pain and taking pain medication, while medication can reduce and dull pain, it may also dull a patients entire system, physically and mentally. This can include a their ability to think, process information, react, communicate, remember things and move around.

During this time, it can be helpful to adjust your energy level to match theirs. For example, if you are a high-energy person, you may need to consciously walk and move a little slower, speak a little slower and quieter and allow more time for a response when asking questions or assisting patients with a task. As the patient heals, their energy and ability to process information will increase, but in the beginning, matching their pace and timing will help you both.

ARE YOU A TOUGH GUY?

It's a funny question, but I've resembled this remark. Some patients like to be tough and stoic, "I'm okay, it doesn't hurt that much," while others may be concerned about the toxic nature and addictive properties of pain medications. Admittedly, I can be stubborn at times and try to tough it out, but please, feel free to learn from my mistakes. On more occasions than I'd like to admit, I have waited too long to take pain medication and have ended up in excruciating pain, which caused unnecessary suffering.

Staying ahead of pain is key.

Taking prescription pain medication as prescribed can help keep pain under control, support rest and allow healing to commence. Once pain spikes, it can be hard to get it back under control. Chasing pain or being on a pain rollercoaster increases stress and burns energy that could be better channeled into healing. Pain and pain rollercoasters may also magnify any challenges you may be experiencing or facing and zap patience. A regular pain management schedule, recommended by your doctor, can be really helpful. It is not for forever, but rather a tool to get you through a rough patch.

If you're experiencing pain, be sure to clearly communicate this to your doctor so appropriate measures to alleviate it can be taken. Everyone's tolerance to pain medication is different. Some people's bodies are extremely sensitive to medications and others are not. *If you're experiencing significant pain, your doctor needs to know.*

THE MOST EFFECTIVE PAIN MANAGEMENT PLAN INCLUDES:

- **Communicating with your doctor about your pain**
- **Staying on top of post-surgical pain**
- **Being flexible to make adjustments along the way**

Everyone's tolerance to pain and pain medication is different.
Pain management is not an exact science;
it's a process that may require adjusting along the way.

TRACK YOUR PAIN: CAUSES, INTENSITY, INTERVENTION, EFFECTIVENESS

Tracking pain (using a traditional 0-10 scale—"no pain" to "worst imaginable pain") and what you do that alleviates pain can be helpful in managing it.

Make notes on pain intensity, activities that increase (or decrease) pain and what you did to manage pain (such as what medication you took or which technique you used), and its effectiveness. Use the template on page 184 to track your pain.

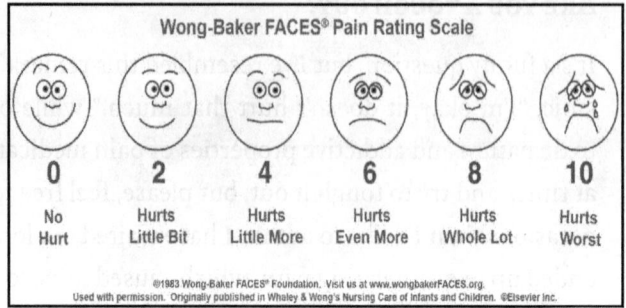

Wong-Baker FACES® Pain Rating Scale

0	2	4	6	8	10
No Hurt	Hurts Little Bit	Hurts Little More	Hurts Even More	Hurts Whole Lot	Hurts Worst

©1983 Wong-Baker FACES® Foundation. Visit us at www.wongbakerFACES.org.
Used with permission. Originally published in Whaley & Wong's Nursing Care of Infants and Children. ©Elsevier Inc.

Following my head injury, pain management templates were incredibly helpful to me and my doctor as we worked together to manage my pain. They were also a wonderful resource for me to witness my improvement. When I felt like I was never going to get any better, I could look back at all the progress I had made. I had evidence that I was, in fact, getting better overall, even if it didn't feel that way in that moment.

OTHER PAIN MANAGEMENT TOOLS

As each body is unique, so, too, is each individual's tolerance and experience of pain. While acute post-surgical pain is most commonly treated with pain medication prescribed by your doctor, there are many ways—both traditional and complementary tools and techniques—to manage pain. (Pages 63-66 discuss traditional pain management tools and techniques and pages 67-71 discuss complementary pain management tools and techniques.) Traditional and complementary techniques have been shown to work well both independently and together. I found that a combination worked best for me. You will need to be the judge as to what is right for you.

TRADITIONAL PAIN MANAGEMENT TOOLS AND TECHNIQUES

MODERN PHARMACEUTICALS

The use of modern pharmaceuticals, such as Dilaudid, Morphine, Oxycontin, Vicodin (a combination of hydrocodone and acetaminophen[xi]), Vicoprofen (a combination of hydrocodone and ibuprofen), Percocet, Ultracet and others is usually a doctor's traditional first approach to managing pain.

There are pluses and minuses to this approach. The upside of pain medication is that it can provide relief when you need it. One of the down sides is that pain medication, especially opiates and opiate-based medications, can also have a variety of side or "other" effects. Depending on the drug(s) you're prescribed, and your unique physique and body chemistry, these *"other effects"* can have a wide range of symptoms.

Sometimes pain medication can cause or deepen emotional side effects. Opiates specifically can have a depressant effect on the central nervous system, which can negatively impact the mind and emotions. Some pain medications can also cause memory gaps or even erase memory.[xii]

Each patient will have a different experience. Some may experience one or two side effects while others may experience several side effects varying in intensity from mild to serious.

A list of side or other effects from pain medications can be found on page 64. This list isn't intended to alarm you, but rather to make you aware of possible effects you may experience.[xiii] If you experience adverse side effects, speak with your doctor so that together you can devise a pain solution that works for you without creating more problems.

[xi] Some are more familiar with acetaminophen's brand name, Tylenol.

[xii] This is also the case with a group of drugs called benzodiazepines (also known as "benzos"), such as Xanax, or the more powerful Versed (usually used just before and during surgery), which are used to cause relaxation and sleepiness. They are known to cause partial to complete loss of memory.

[xiii] Other prescription or over-the-counter medications you may be taking (including some vitamins, herbs or recreational drugs) may interact with pain medications, either heightening or diminishing their effects. To avoid negative drug reactions, inform your doctor of all medications or natural products you are taking.

"SIDE EFFECTS"—OTHER EFFECTS—THAT MAY BE CAUSED BY PAIN MEDICATION:

Call or see your doctor immediately if any of the following SERIOUS effects occur:

- Allergic reactions: swelling of the face, lips, tongue or throat, hives, difficult or labored breathing
- Altered mental state, hallucinations
- Paranoia
- Hyperventilation
- Seizures or convulsions

Other possible effects include:

- Constipation
- Dizziness, light-headedness or feeling like you might pass out
- Nausea, upset stomach or vomiting
- Decreased or loss of appetite
- Dry mouth
- Itching, warmth, tingling or redness under the skin
- Sweating or hot flashes
- Muscle twitching
- Headaches
- Memory problems (may forget things such as conversations or visits)
- Depression, despair, hopelessness
- Anxiety
- Agitation, frustration, irritability
- Emotional, moody
- Confusion, indecisiveness
- Slowness, fuzziness
- Unusual fatigue/tired feeling
- Sleep problems, such as insomnia or the opposite, sleeping too much
- Diminished sex drive or loss of interest in sex
- Unusual thoughts or behavior
- Severe weakness
- Possible long-term addiction

For me, prescription pain medications have helped alleviate some pain when I needed it, but the negative for me was that I felt they contributed to blue feelings, dry mouth, constipation, memory problems and some moodiness. If you notice undesirable effects from doctor prescribed pain management medication, talk to your doctor about it. Some solutions may include:

- **Adjusting medications**
- **Trying a different medication.** There are many pain management drug categories. If one doesn't work well for you, there may be an alternative solution available.
- **Examining and trying alternatives to taking the medication altogether**

Pain medications also can be addictive, even when taken exactly as prescribed by your doctor, for even relatively short periods of time. For example, following my open-heart surgery I was on a prescription pain medication for several weeks, tapering the dose as I felt better. The last week I only took a small dose at night to help me sleep. However, when I stopped taking even that small dose, I experienced some symptoms of physical withdrawal: hot and cold flashes, body aches, frustration, moodiness and sleeplessness. Not knowing why I was feeling so poorly, I called and asked my doctor about my symptoms. He confirmed that even though my dose had been small, my body had simply gotten used to—dependent on—the medication and was in fact detoxing and readjusting now that I had stopped.

Ask your doctor questions about drugs being prescribed and what possible short- or long-term effects may exist. It's up to you to really understand the pluses and minuses of medications you are taking so you can make educated decisions about how you want to proceed.

Note: **Pharmacists are a wealth of knowledge and a phenomenal resource** for questions about pain (and other) medications.

Pharmacists are experts in identifying medication side effects and possible drug interactions.

Pharmacists are schooled six-plus years in medicinal chemistry, pathophysiology and pharmacotherapy and must pass national and state licensing exams.

To assist in keeping track of medications and possible interactions, get all your prescriptions filled at one pharmacy.[xiv] I have used the same pharmacy for nearly 15 years. Over time I have gotten to know the pharmacists there and they have been an invaluable resource for me on multiple occasions. I am so grateful and thankful for my pharmacists!

ICE

Applying ice to an incision site causes a reduction in nerve conduction velocity and reduces swelling which can cause pain. (Refer back to page 49 for more on ice and swelling.) Common sense and experience tell us that numbness from icing can also deaden pain.

[xiv] The role a pharmacist plays in patient care is currently undergoing change and is in the process of coming into a new age. This will include a new aspect of care called medication therapy management which is a distinct service or group of services that optimizes drug therapy with the intent of improved therapeutic outcomes for individual patients. Medication therapy management is a unique niche for the pharmacy profession, allowing pharmacists to apply their extensive medication knowledge as "medication experts" with the intent of improving patient outcomes.

ELEVATION

Elevating the surgical site above the heart, if possible, helps blood flow away from the incision and surgical site. This may help alleviate some swelling, throbbing and pain.

PHYSICAL THERAPY

When appropriate, ultrasound, electronic stimulation, exercise and other techniques performed by a physical therapist can help in reducing or relieving pain and promote the healing process. (See pages 92-93 for more on physical therapy and physical therapy tools.) Physical therapy is prescribed by your doctor.

TIME

Day by day, week by week, month by month and year after year the body continues to heal; it's always working, whether we're thinking about it or not. If your pain is estimated to decrease over a three-week period, the only way to get from day one to day 21 is one day at a time. This is where patience comes into play.

Complementary Pain Management Tools and Techniques

While most people have heard the term "alternative medicine," the term *complementary medicine* is more accurate. Complementary medicine is not an alternative to medical care or recommendations made by your doctor, but rather is intended to complement what your doctor is doing.

What is complementary medicine?

The field of complementary medicine is vast and exciting. It encompasses both the leading edge of science and ancient healing traditions, including those from China and India. Closer to home, the ancient cultures throughout the Americas also have extensive healing traditions. Complementary medicine can be brilliant and filled with incredible solutions that sadly haven't yet been investigated, let alone been approved, by the U.S. Food and Drug Administration (FDA).

I have used complementary techniques successfully both in conjunction with traditional pain management techniques and independently. For me, incorporating complementary medicine into my recoveries has been a positive experience. I believe it has contributed to quicker easier post-surgical recoveries for me. However, it is up to you to explore and see what is right for you. The following are a few ideas.

Meditation

There is a great deal of scientific and medical research confirming that meditation reduces pain perception and aids in healing. Research has revealed that Zen meditators have lower pain sensitivity both in and out of a meditative state compared to non-meditators.[6] In one published study, Zen meditators experienced an 18% reduction in pain intensity. Moreover, when control subjects were instructed and practiced meditation for five months, their brain response to pain decreased by 40-50%.[7,8] Even beginners have success alleviating pain with meditation.[9] I personally have found meditation effective in shifting my mind away from pain back to the present moment. Meditation is one of the oldest methods of relaxation. The action of achieving a state of relaxation or awareness brings about a peaceful frame of mind and a state of calm.

While many books have been written on the subject, meditation can be as simple as sitting quietly and focusing on the breath. For example, next time you inhale and exhale, pay attention to the air moving in and out of your body—in through the nose, out through the mouth. As you do this, you'll notice that thoughts, concerns and the constant chatter taking place in your mind drift away. If the chatter starts back up, stop and refocus your attention back on your breathing. Doing this for just one to two minutes at a time, whenever you think of it, can alleviate anxiety or panic and decrease pain. (See pages 196-197 for meditation and relaxation exercises.)

SCIENTIFIC STUDIES HAVE FOUND MEDITATION:

- **Appears to reduce people's sensitivity to pain**
- **Causes an individual to be less fearful of pain**
- **Useful in reducing the emotional impact of pain**
- **Trains the brain to be more present-focused.** Spending less time anticipating future negative events may be why meditation is effective at reducing the recurrence of depression, which has been associated with making pain worse.
- **Encourages slower, more full, productive breaths**, which can reduce pain
- **Allows the body to rest in a relaxed state**
- **Creates a more balanced outlook on life.** One study suggests that this is not just an attitudinal change, but also a fundamental change in how the brain functions.
- **Increases activity in the parasympathetic nervous system (PNS).** This causes breathing to be deeper and more relaxed and the heart rate to slow, promoting rest.
- **Reduces activity in the sympathetic nervous system (SNS) and triggers the PNS.** The SNS is responsible for the body's the "fight-or-flight response" which causes the heart rate to increase, breathing to be more rapid, but shallow, and blood flow to be diverted away from the organs, to the extremities, causing people to tense their muscles. This response is helpful in an emergency, but counterproductive in alleviating pain and healing.[10]

DEEP BREATHING AND BREATH WORK

Breathing for pain control? Absolutely.
Ask any mother who's experienced a natural childbirth.

Oxygen is important. The human body can go for extended periods of time without food or water, but only a few minutes without oxygen. As a pain management technique, studies (and my own personal experiences) have found that deep breathing techniques can help with pain, anxiety and stress before and after a medical procedure, or any time.

Also known as diaphragmatic, controlled or purposeful breathing, it works by disengaging the body's natural automatic response to any painful, stressful or tense situation, which is to hold our breath. A quick, shallow breath automatically follows shock or pain. However, continuing to hold our breath deprives the brain and body of oxygen (fuel), which can exacerbate pain. It's very difficult to hold your breath and release tension at the same time, which is why sighing is so important.

Deep breathing also clears out carbon dioxide and increases oxygen. Shallow breathing does just the opposite.

To gain the benefits of deep breathing, take slow, measured, rhythmic deep breaths. Be sure to inhale deeply, into your belly (not just your chest). Watch the abdomen expand with each inhale and completely deflate with each exhale.

CONSCIOUSLY TAKING SLOW, DEEP, MEASURED, CLEANSING BREATHS CAN HELP:

- **Relax muscles**
- **Calm the mind**
- **Increase oxygen to cells**
- **Encourage the production and release of endorphins**, the body's natural painkillers
- **Clear the mind**. A clear mind can make healthy, proactive choices.
- **Avoid panic or fear-driven actions** often caused by pain

MASSAGE THERAPY AND BODYWORK

Chinese medical literature describes the traditional use of massage and bodywork in healing for over 4,000 years. Within the field of massage therapy there exists a wide array of techniques and touch therapies that can be wonderful tools to support and assist the body (and the mind) in healing, pain relief and recovery. Receiving bodywork after surgery can contribute to the healing process.

Note: There are instances where, following surgery, massage therapy may be contraindicated such as in the presence of an infection, open wound or blood clot. Check with your doctor first. (See pages 192-194 for information on some specific massage therapy techniques.)

THE BENEFITS OF MASSAGE THERAPY

Even a light, or short, massage can assist body functions and facilitate healing and recovery, physically, emotionally and mentally by:

- **Stimulating the immune system** which has been shown to help reduce or prevent post-surgical infections
- **Increasing blood flow and circulation** which can assist the body in flushing toxins, reduce swelling and improve the flow of nutrients to injured areas
- **Promoting parasympathetic responses** which can alleviate spasms and cramping
- **Stimulating the nervous system** which is known to boost energy and provide relaxation, reducing depression and anxiety
- **Stimulating and releasing endorphins**, the body's natural painkillers
- **Regenerating tissue** around wounds and reducing or preventing scar tissue
- **Assisting elimination** by relaxing abdominal and intestinal muscles

ACUPUNCTURE

Originating over 3,000 years ago in China, acupuncture is an ancient health care system based on the concept that energy (also known as qi or chi) flows through the body in certain patterns (meridians). There are 365 main points along 12 primary meridians which when stimulated relieve a wide range of symptoms and conditions. If there is a blockage or imbalance in the meridian system it can lead to pain, congestion or disease (dis-ease).

Acupuncture identifies blockages. By inserting fine needles into specific points along the meridian paths, the practitioner releases energy blockages and energizes or tonifies deficiencies. Acupuncture has also been shown to release endorphins which relieve pain, balance moods and pain perception, enhance recuperative powers, strengthen the immune system and promote well-being.

HYPNOTHERAPY

For acute pain, hypnosis has been shown to be effective in the treatment of various surgical procedures, bone marrow aspiration, burns, dental work, childbirth labor and other pain.[11] Some reports state that with hypnosis, the need for standard narcotic pain intervention also decreases.[12] Hypnosis has also been used successfully in treating chronic pain conditions including headaches, backaches, carcinoma-related pain, fibromyalgia, temporal mandibular pain and mixed chronic pain.

Hypnosis is a growing field and today there continues to be a lot of research in this area for both acute and chronic pain. One variance linked to the success of hypnosis has to do with the quality of the practitioner and the posthypnotic suggestions given to a patient. Different posthypnotic suggestions may elicit different degrees of relief.

ENERGY WORK

Some people find relief using energy techniques such as Reiki, Therapeutic Touch or Crystalline Consciousness Technique which work with the body's energy systems to balance physical, mental and emotional well-being and promote a state of deep relaxation. With her over 30 years in the healing arts, gia combs-ramirez has consistently found that when you, "take care of the energy, healing follows with grace and ease."[13] Energy healing is particularly helpful in working with emotional and mental traumas, conditions that affect the central nervous system, PTSD, sensory dysfunction and chronic viral issues. (See page 195 for more information on energy work techniques.)

Sleeping and Resting

. . .

Sleeping and resting following surgery are paramount for healing and recovery. Sleep and rest create and support the foundation for ongoing optimal health: physically, mentally and emotionally. While they may seem similar, they are different, but equally valuable.

Sleeping

Prior to surgery, good sleep can help build energy reserves. Following surgery, your body will be expending greater amounts of energy than normal due to stress, anxiety, pain and healing. Energy and energy reserves can quickly become exhausted. Sound, solid, deep, restorative sleep is crucial in healing.

There are five stages of sleep (four levels and REM). The most significant time your body releases somatotropin, the regenerative growth hormone required for healing, is when the body reaches deep stage three and stage four sleep.

Lack of sleep can impede healing, alter mood, cause irritability and lessen your ability to cope with stress. It can also exacerbate pain, put you at a risk of depression and impair focus, concentration and memory.

Lack of sleep slows down everything.

Sometimes sleeping after surgery can be difficult or disturbed by pain, discomfort and anxiety. If you're in the hospital, additional disruptions may include nurses administering medications, aides checking vital signs, loud unfamiliar noises and insufficient darkness.

If you're in a noisy hospital or rehabilitation center or your home environment is loud, use earplugs. If it's bright, shut off the lights, pull the curtains and put on a sleep mask. Filter out noise and light so you can rest. While sleep disturbances are normal following surgery, it is important for the body to rest so it can heal.

If you're having trouble sleeping:

- **Take pain medication ½ hour before bedtime**
- **Avoid caffeine in the afternoon and evening**

IF THAT DOESN'T WORK:

- **Look at your diet**. (See pages 85-86 for specific suggestions on "good" and "bad" foods for promoting a restful night's sleep.)
- **Try a warm relaxing bath or shower before bed**, if possible
- **Get into a regular bedtime routine**. A consistent routine will let your body know it's time to relax and go to sleep.
- **Ask someone to give you a back or foot rub**. As a child, when I couldn't sleep, my dad would rub my back. It always worked like a charm; sound asleep in no time.
- **Empty your brain**. If your mind is abuzz at bedtime, take a minute to write down all the thoughts, feelings, worries and fears running around in your head. This accomplishes two things: (1) now you have a list of things to tackle the next day and (2) your brain can now rest, knowing everything has been safely written down, where it can be accessed later.
- **Avoid television and computers before bedtime**. Watching television or working at the computer can be stimulating and may prevent melatonin levels from rising to induce sleep. Graphic violence, especially at bedtime, can also cause anxiety levels to rise, negatively affecting sleep.
- **Listen to relaxing music or a guided imagery audio program**
- **Read**
- **Exercise during the day**. If your physician clears it, add some exercise into your routine. Start with light exercise and gradually increase. Try 20-30 minutes a day, to begin. If necessary, break 20-30 minute blocks down even further into 10-minute sessions. (Read more about the benefits of exercise on pages 95-96.)
- **Try a simple self-relaxation technique such as progressive muscle relaxation**. (See pages 196-197 for simple and effective exercises.)

UGH, NOTHING'S WORKING!

If none of the previous suggestions help and you're not getting a good solid night's rest, it may be time to speak with your doctor about some kind of temporary intervention that will: (1) assist you in getting to sleep and (2) hold you at a deep level three/level four restorative sleep. Lack of sleep following surgery can have some immediate consequences such as slowed healing, unchecked emotions, irritability, impaired cognitive function, loss of balance, headaches, memory problems and more.

▪ ▪ ▪

RESTING AND CONSERVING ENERGY

When body motions and functions slow down, rest naturally occurs.

"I'M SO TIRED"

This is totally normal following any surgery, trauma, injury or illness. Even though you may be feeling better, you may tire more quickly and easily or your energy level may be difficult to sustain, even doing previously simple tasks such as showering, washing your hair, preparing and eating a meal, doing a quick errand, or visiting with a friend. While this is to be expected, it can still be frustrating. It's worthwhile to remember: your body has been through a tremendous amount, the physical assault from surgery itself as well as the physical, mental and emotional stress from healing. It takes a great deal of energy for the body to heal itself. As the body funnels energy into healing, it borrows from and depletes its usual pool of energy reserves, possibly leaving you more tired than usual.

Depending on the extent of your surgical procedure, it can take months for the body and its systems to return to "normal." Pushing the body too hard too soon can exhaust it, possibly hampering healing and recovery. Rest and intentional built-in periods of rest can support healing and recovery. This is a good time to be extra kind and patient with yourself, you're healing.

HEALTH CARE SYSTEM CHANGES CAUSE PATIENTS TO BE DISCHARGED SOONER

Due to changes in the health care and insurance systems, patients are spending significantly less time in hospitals following procedures and more time recovering at home. While being at home can be quieter and more relaxing in some ways (no one checking your vitals or asking a bunch of questions every two hours), home recovery can have its own challenges. At home, the tendency may be to do too much, too soon, and not rest as you might in a more isolated hospital setting; there can be a lot of stimulation and distractions from kids, pets and the "to do" list. These are great items to ask for help and support with so you can allow your body the rest it needs to heal. (Refer back to pages 11-17 on support.)

It's helpful to remember that just because you've been discharged from a hospital doesn't mean you're "all better," it just means you are stable enough to continue your recovery at home. It's a process. Let your body be your guide. Be prepared and willing to be a patient patient.

USE YOUR ENERGY WISELY

During the weeks and months following surgery allocate your energy carefully and conserve it for healing where and whenever possible. This can be tricky, because as you begin to feel better, your mind starts "biting off" more than perhaps the body can "chew."

If you're experiencing limited energy, notice where you're expending energy and ask yourself, "is this really what I want to spend my energy on right now?" Be aware that doing a "quick" errand, for example, may require several steps, such as getting out of bed, getting dressed, preparing and eating something, brushing your teeth, brushing your hair, walking to the car, driving, parking, etc., which can, themselves, be tiring. (While you heal, these may also take more time than usual—sometimes, a lot more.)

Fatigue and feeling drained can also be side effects from pain (or other) medications, or it can be from lack of a good night's sleep. Listen to your body. For a period of time following surgery it is likely you will need more rest than a normal night's sleep provides. You may notice that you also need more quiet or alone time. Accept this new—albeit temporary—circumstance and if you feel tired, take note. Allow yourself to slow down or stop whenever necessary.

A friend of mine who had a thoracotomy (which means part of her lung was removed) says, "There is no such thing as 'too much' rest when you are healing!" I would agree.

TIPS AND TOOLS FOR ENERGY CONSERVATION WHILE YOU'RE RECOVERING

As you recuperate, allow yourself and healing to become your number one priority. In the short term, simplify and eliminate unnecessary tasks when possible. Conserved energy is better channeled into healing and recovery. I've learned the hard way that in the end, most things don't really matter. What does matter is you, your recovery, your health and well-being. Here are some energy conservation tips.

- **Ask for help. Avoid unadvised movements such as bending, lifting, leaning, reaching, twisting, walking, or prolonged sitting and standing**. Have someone else get the pot roast out of the oven, take a box to the garage, get a sweater from under the bed, drop off or pick up the dry cleaning or put paper in the copy machine at work.
- **Take your time**. Spread tasks out and allow yourself more time than usual for what-ever you're doing. Avoid rushing or attempting to get things done at your usual pace.

- **Limit visitors or social activities**. While the idea of visitors may feel good, visitors and social activities can be draining. (Note: Even fun, seemingly easy activities such as a visit from, or lunch with, a close friend can be an exhausting, draining activity, but not to worry, your energy and stamina will return in time.)

- **Set realistic goals and priorities**. Ask yourself, "What are today's *real* priorities?" Before taking action, pause and check in with yourself, see what your body has to say. In this moment, is taking action in your highest and best good? Be prepared and allow yourself to change course if your body sends you a "no."

- **Create a list and organize it for efficiency** to avoid unnecessary running around.

- **Avoid long lists and allow for the possibility that not everything may get accomplished**. I've learned from experience that the sky doesn't fall if everything on my list doesn't get done; it just gets moved to another list for another day when I have more energy. Give yourself permission to stop, rest or go back to bed if necessary.

- **Don't start an activity that can't be stopped**. If you start an involved project, give yourself permission, ahead of time, to leave it incomplete if you begin to feel tired.

- **Stop an activity *before* you get tired**. It will be there later; you can come back to it.

- **Take catnaps**. Consciously and intentionally scheduling periods of rest—lying down and napping for 15-30 minutes between activities—can make a difference.

EATING AND DRINKING TO SUPPORT HEALING AND RECOVERY

■ ■ ■

What we eat and drink directly impacts our health and well-being on all levels. Nutrition—a proper diet—is paramount for success in day-to-day life, but especially so when preparing for and recovering from the effects of surgery. Without food and water, we will die. Beyond that, what we eat and drink, how much and when, can help shape healing and recovery.

Food and the nutrients it provides is the fuel that feeds every cell and every system in the body; affecting all its components: physical, mental and emotional. Following the trauma of surgery, when the body has been physically cut into, replenishing and fueling these systems is more important than ever. Good nutrient-dense food provides the essential building blocks to fuel healing and recovery. While surgery can use up significantly more energy and nutrients than normal and slow us down, healthy eating can get us back on our feet and move recovery forward.

WHAT I THINK

I am passionate about food and eating to support my body and mind and I have experienced awesome results with healing, health and wellness from adjusting my diet. I am also fortunate to have had great coaching over the years from family practice physician Todd Mangum, M.D. His approach to medicine and healing is based on what the body needs to heal and function optimally. What I've learned from him about all things diet and food related has helped me make better choices, which has kept me healthier overall and helped me successfully heal from injuries and surgery.

Thanks to this education and greater understanding of food, I have become much more conscious of what I put in my mouth. I have increased my consumption of fresh foods and eliminated most processed foods from my diet. It has made a world of difference in my energy level, stamina, emotional health, mental clarity and overall well-being.

When I think about food, I think about the fact that whatever I put in my mouth gets broken down by my digestive system and distributed throughout my entire body, feeding each cell and driving each system. I can be very pragmatic about food—it's like putting gas in a car. Put sugar in a gas tank and the system is shot. Fill it with high-grade fuel and it will get me to where I want to go. Weighing the pros and cons of a snack, for example, will often lead me to a high-protein snack, which I know will give me energy and get me where I want to go. A half dozen cookies or a muffin (even a bran muffin) loaded with refined flour and sugar will render the opposite effect, leaving me jittery, anxious, unfocused and less productive.

So, I use food to heal and feel better. After surgery I want to get back on my feet and back to doing what I love. (See example on page 94.) Eating well is a tool to get me there. Having said that, what I believe to be true about food may be very different than what someone else believes. My intention here is to bring some awareness to foods that can positively contribute to healing and recovery.

THE DARK SIDE

Over the years, as I have become more aware, I have become deeply disappointed with the bags of rubbish that food and beverage manufacturers have sold to me and other trusting consumers. In my opinion, manufacturers have become deceitful and manipulative in the name of profits. They make products with endless health claims filled with inexpensive, unhealthy, addictive ingredients including hydrogenated fats and preservatives to extend their shelf life, all at the cost of our health. Many of these "foods" are carefully engineered with just the right mix of sugars, trans-fats and chemicals to keep us consuming them in vast quantities and coming back for more.

This is an area where we as individuals can step up and assume more responsibility.

WHAT IS A HEALTHY DIET?

According to Dr. Mangum,

> *"A healthy diet is one that makes you feel good all day long.*
> *It is one that digests easily and comfortably.*
> *A healthy diet will help you maintain or regain vibrant health and well-being."*

Unfortunately, some people don't eat well when they don't feel well. However, not eating can actually make patients feel worse. Patients can also lose their appetite or feel nauseated from pain or medications, especially if taken on an empty stomach. If you're feeling nauseated after surgery, begin slowly, eating what you can. Start with small nutritious meals or snacks and build up as you feel better. While some foods provide more nutrients than others, in some cases, when a patient doesn't feel well, simply eating anything may be all that is possible at the time.

Healthy, nutrient-rich food can positively impact your recovery by:

- Providing the necessary building blocks your skin and body need to heal
- Improving and speeding wound healing
- Generating energy
- Supporting emotional health and fostering feelings of well-being
- Limiting some complications, such as constipation. (See pages 51-57 on constipation.)
- Assisting with a good night's sleep. (See pages 72-76 on sleeping and resting.)

Are there right—or wrong—things to eat before and after surgery?

In a word, yes. The same foods that are good for healing before and after surgery are the same foods that are healthy to eat all the time.

Eating real whole foods fuels the body with nutrients for healing

One of the best things you can do to supply your body with the vitamins, minerals and nutrients it needs to heal is to eat real, whole, nutrient-dense foods. This means choosing natural, unprocessed (or minimally processed) foods, rather than boxed, canned or frozen versions.

The easiest way to find fresh nutrient-dense foods at the market is to do your grocery shopping in the outer ring of the supermarket, not within the aisles. Most grocery stores are set up with fresh vegetables, fruits, meat, fish, eggs and dairy products in the store's periphery.[xv] Canned, packaged and highly processed foods line the shelves of the inner aisles. Shopping around the aisles, you will naturally find more nutritious foods. This applies to health food stores as well. Granted, the food found in health food stores will generally be of better quality and contain fewer unhealthy ingredients compared to products found in commercial grocery stores. However, even health food stores stock their aisles with landmines of sugar- and carbohydrate-laden products.

Examples of real—whole—foods and why they are a better choice

Take an orange; it's a whole food. Orange juice, on the other hand, unless you squeeze it yourself, is processed. During processing and pasteurizing, natural vitamins and minerals are lost.

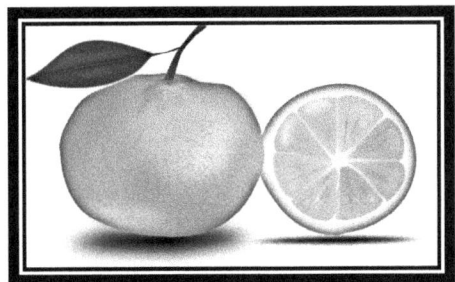

[xv] The exception to this rule is the bakery, which is also usually found in the supermarket periphery.

A whole orange is a better choice because in addition to the natural vitamins and minerals found in the juice, you also get valuable fiber and roughage from the pulp and innards. The fiber from an orange is beneficial because it: (1) aids in digestion, (2) supports reduction of harmful cholesterol and (3) helps balance blood sugars, keeping them from dramatically spiking from the natural sugar found in the juice. Eating oranges versus drinking juice will also aid you in feeling fuller and more satisfied, helping to eliminate overeating. It is much less likely that you will consume the same amount of fruit that you can easily drink when it's juiced. When was the last time you sat and ate six oranges in under 30 seconds? Easy to do with a glass of juice, but near impossible with the whole fruit. The same is true with apples and apple juice and so on.

Another example: a baked potato (with the skin on). Even covered in butter (which is a healthy fat), cheese, sour cream and chives, is a far healthier choice than boxed mashed potatoes or fast food French fries. Both highly processed alternatives provide little to no nutritional value. Boxed mashed potatoes contain significantly more sodium than fresh potatoes and less dietary fiber, vitamin C, protein, vitamins and minerals. Some boxed potatoes, such as "Betty Crocker Roasted Garlic Potatoes made with 100% real mashed potatoes seasoned with roasted garlic," also contain added sugar, monosodium glutamate (MSG, a flavor enhancer known to trigger headaches and other adverse reactions), partially hydrogenated oil (trans-fat), artificial flavor and artificial color. Most fast food French fries are basically starch cooked in rancid fat and then loaded with salt.[14]

PROCESSED, PACKAGED AND FAST FOODS

Processed, packaged foods have almost completely taken over the American diet. Unfortunately, most processed foods are laden with sugar, high-fructose corn syrup, salt[xvi], artificial sweeteners (such as aspartame), artificial flavors (such as MSG), artificial colors, factory-created trans-fats (hydrogenated and partially hydrogenated fats and oils), preservatives and other chemicals that alter food nutrition, texture and flavor. The trouble is not just what's been added to processed food, but also with what's been taken away. Processed foods are often stripped of nutrients and healthy fats.[15]

[xvi] Approximately three-quarters of the sodium we ingest is from processed and packaged goods, not from salt added to food at the dinner table. Salt is hidden in canned vegetables and soups, condiments, fast foods and cured and preserved meats.

PRODUCT NAMES, LABELS AND LABEL READING

In today's world of marketing and advertising, even a product's name is suspect. To really know what exactly a product does—or does not—contain, consumers must carefully read the ingredient list. For example, just because bread is called whole wheat doesn't mean it's not loaded with other poor ingredients, nor does it even indicate what percentage of the flour is whole wheat. Ignore claims printed on the front of food packaging. The trick is to go straight to the ingredient label on the back where fortunately, by law, companies have to list everything in their product. This is where you will find out what a product really contains.

HOW DOES ONE MAKE GOOD CHOICES?

If you are overwhelmed by the number of ingredients in a product, especially those you cannot pronounce, a simple rule to begin with is: Don't eat it if you don't know what it is. Becoming aware of what ingredients make up a product is the first step and educating yourself about those ingredients is the next. I can get so frustrated when I read labels with their confusing list of ingredients.

Learning about food and ingredients in packaged foods and making choices is a process. Rather than becoming overwhelmed, I simply make the best choices I can with the information I have. What I've found is that as I become more educated, my choices continue to evolve. Sometimes it's not about making the "perfect" choice, but about simply making a "better" choice.

ORGANIC. HOW IS IT DIFFERENT? WHY IS IT BETTER?

The question of organic comes up a lot and many are confused as to if, or why, it's better. What does organic mean? The Merriam-Webster dictionary defines organic as,

> *"of food: grown or made without the use of artificial chemicals;*
> *of, relating to, or obtained from living things."*

Simply, yes, organic is better. Here's why: Organic meat, dairy and produce cannot contain any unnatural chemicals such as pesticides, herbicides, fungicides or synthetic fertilizers, nitrates, preservatives, growth hormones or antibiotics or be genetically modified (GMO). I believe this is important to know, because when ingested, these toxic chemical and artificial ingredients must be processed by the body, which can be exceptionally taxing to a system which is already taxed from surgery and the enormous amount of energy it takes to heal.

Is it all or nothing?

Faced with all the information out there, eating organic doesn't have to be all or nothing. Start simple. For example, consider purchasing vegetables and fruit with skins that come directly into contact with pesticides and herbicides organically grown and purchase items that have an outer layer that can be peeled away conventionally grown. For me, while my preference is all-organic all the time, sometimes I must choose. In this case I'd choose the following produce:

Organically Grown		Conventionally Grown*	
Apples	Nectarines & peaches	Avocado	Oranges
Blueberries	Potatoes	Bananas	Papayas
Celery	Spinach & greens	Cabbage	Pineapples
Cherries	Strawberries	Cantaloupe	Sweet peas
Cucumber	Tomatoes	Eggplant	Tangerines
Grapes	Zucchini	Grapefruit	Watermelon

*Conventionally grown choices have a thick outer skin that can be peeled away.

We must become champions and advocates for our own health and well-being in whatever way corresponds with our personal values. Review available information and then make choices that work for you. For me, it continues to be an ongoing process and education.

So, what does work?
What foods should I focus on following surgery?

First, pay attention to and listen to your body. If you're having trouble with energy, inflammation, gas, aches, pains, weakness, sleep, anxiety or other symptoms, take note and look at your diet. What are you eating and drinking and when? Then, play with your food. Adjust, limit or eliminate foods such as sugar, grains, dairy, meat and carbonated sodas and add healthy protein (chicken, fish, tofu, nuts), good fats (butter, olive oil, coconut oil, lard), fresh vegetables and fresh fruits and more water. Try eating smaller meals more frequently. See if you notice a difference. Do you feel better?

Eating for health and healing is about eating and drinking
what we know works nutritionally and chemically for the human body.

THE HUMAN BODY USES **PROTEIN** AS BUILDING BLOCKS.
PROTEIN CAN ALSO BE CONVERTED TO FUEL.

Protein is necessary to build and repair blood, bones, muscles, cartilage, skin and hair; manufacture antibodies to protect the body and fight disease and illness; make hormones and other necessary body chemicals; transmit signals between cells, tissues and organs; and support the liver and its detoxification pathways.

CARBOHYDRATES PROVIDE ENERGY FOR NORMAL BODY FUNCTIONS

Carbohydrates provide energy for our heartbeat, breathing, digestion and brain activity. They also support daily activities such as walking, climbing stairs, exercise and healing. What many people are confused about is where to obtain healthy carbohydrates. The best most nutritious carbohydrates are obtained from vegetables and fruits. Vegetables are the best because they don't spike blood sugar or insulin and they are packed with fiber and nutrients.

THE CONSUMPTION OF GOOD **FATS** PROMOTES GOOD HEALTH

The body requires healthy fat in the diet to function optimally. After surgery, this means healing. While fats are a complex topic, the thing to remember is fat is not the enemy, but synthetic trans-fats (hydrogenated or partially hydrogenated fats and oils) artificially created in laboratories as cheaper alternatives to butter, are![xvii] Butter, coconut oil, olive oil and even lard are considered good fats, as are coconut milk, avocado and nuts. In moderation, healthy sources of fat can assist with digestion, elimination, metabolism and mood regulation; protect tissues and organs; contribute to better sleep; stabilize blood sugar; reduce inflammation; regulate "good" and "bad" cholesterols; and more.

Important members of this family are essential fatty acids (EFAs) which cannot be produced by the body or converted from other fats in the body. EFAs must be obtained through the diet. Omega-3s and omega-6s in balance are vital for good health. Omega-3s are important because of their many benefits including healthier, stronger bones, protection of tissues and organs from inflammation and help with mood regulation. However, according to Dr. Mangum, while most people are lacking in omega-3s, most people get an overabundance of omega-6s. One consequence of too much omega-6 is that it can increase inflammation in the body.

[xvii] In November 2013, even the FDA came out against hydrogenated and partially hydrogenated oils. "Reducing trans-fat intake could prevent thousands of heart attacks and deaths... Partially hydrogenated oils, the primary dietary source of artificial *trans*-fat in processed foods, are not generally recognized as safe for use in food." Yet, hydrogenated and partially hydrogenated fats and oils remain as ingredients and additives in thousands of foods.

One reason for the unintentional overconsumption of omega-6 fatty acids is because omega-6 fatty acids are found in abundance in vegetable oils which are used excessively in processed foods (sunflower oil, corn oil, soybean oil, cottonseed oil, canola oil and peanut oil). Even health foods contain vegetable oils, which is another reason it is crucial to read ingredient labels. (The widespread use of vegetable oil in cooking has risen dramatically over the last one hundred years, which is why we tend to consume significantly more omega-6s than omega-3s.)

Good sources of omega-3 fatty acids include hemp, flax and chia seeds, walnuts, leafy greens, algae, fish and fish oil supplements. (Note: Omega-3 essential fatty acids are especially fragile and should *always* be refrigerated. Fish oil, flaxseeds and hemp seeds, among others, should always be kept in the refrigerator as they will oxidize and become toxic and rancid if they are exposed to light, heat or air.)

HOSPITAL FOOD

If you're in the hospital, you may want to ask visitors to bring you something nutritious to eat (noting, of course, any dietary restraints).

> *"Perhaps the hospital's most serious failure was in the area of nutrition. It was not just that the meals were poorly balanced; what seemed inexcusable to me was the profusion of processed foods, some of which contained preservatives or harmful dyes. White bread, with its chemical softeners and bleached flour, was offered with every meal. Vegetables were often over-cooked and thus deprived of much of their nutritional value."[16]*
>
> Norman Cousins, author, Anatomy of An Illness

Sadly, hospital food hasn't improved much since 1979 when this was written. Processed foods have become even more prevalent in hospital food and our daily diet.

CONSEQUENCES

The consequences are simple,

You are what you eat.

One key to nutritious eating is to be sure your kitchen is stocked with nutritious foods.

Quick Tips and Insights

Food and mood: Good food = good mood!

A healthy diet can help fight depression. Here are some quick tips:

- **Eat more mood-stabilizing foods like protein and fresh vegetables.**
- **Up your intake of omega-3 fatty acids.** These facilitate the brain's "feel good" neurotransmitters, serotonin and dopamine.
- **Limit sugar.** Sugar interferes with brain chemistry, causing a drop in serotonin after the sugar high wears off.
- **Limit junk food.** These have been shown to cause inflammation and to negatively affect brain chemistry.
- **Drink more water.** The brain is made up of electrical circuits and water is the conductor that bridges these circuits. Without enough water, brain signals get dropped, thoughts get cut short and memory can go on the fritz, which can lead to feeling slow, unproductive and blue—disconnected.

Food and constipation: Ingredients likely to worsen constipation

- **Processed, frozen, boxed or canned meals or foods.** These are usually packed with artificial ingredients, hydrogenated and partially hydrogenated oils, sugar, sugar substitutes, refined white flour and white flour products and an overabundance of salt.
- **Fast foods.** Fast foods contain all the above and are low in fiber and other nutrients.
- **Starchy foods**
- **Red meat and pork.** They can be hard to digest and may further slow down the gut, which may already be slow as a result of surgery.
- **Extra spicy food.** Spices such as chili peppers and horseradish can irritate the bowels, contributing to constipation.
- **Coffee, tea and other caffeinated beverages**
- **Alcohol**

Food and sleep

A healthy diet can help with sleep and rest. Here are some quick tips:

- **Avoid caffeine in the afternoon and evening.** Coffee, black tea, colas, "energy" drinks, chocolate, even some over-the-counter headache and pain remedies—such as Excedrin—contain caffeine, a stimulant that can interrupt sleep patterns.

Recommendations: Try soothing, caffeine-free herbal teas. Chamomile is a good choice. Chamomile is used in pharmacopoeia in over 26 countries for its anti-inflammatory, antibacterial, antiallergenic and sedative properties.

- **Eat foods that contain tryptophan before bed.** Tryptophan is the amino acid the body uses to make serotonin, the neurotransmitter that slows down nerve traffic. Try turkey, eggs, chicken, fish, soybeans, tofu, some seeds and nuts.

- **Avoid sugar at bedtime.** Eating sugar causes blood sugar to rise and a corresponding increase in insulin output. This causes blood sugar to drop, releasing adrenalin that can increase anxiety, make you restless and jittery.

- **Have a small, low-glycemic, fat- and protein-rich snack before bedtime.** A snack with protein, fat and little or no sugar will keep blood sugar stable and let adrenal glands know that the body is fed and safe and it's okay to relax and go to sleep. (High-glycemic index snacks, such as ice cream or cookies create the opposite effect.)

Quick and simple low-glycemic bedtime snack ideas:	
Chicken, turkey or tuna	Peanut butter on celery, apples or carrots
Avocado wrapped in a slice of turkey	Almonds or other nuts
Hard-boiled or scrambled egg	Cheese and crackers
A small slice of quiche	Cottage cheese

- **Avoid spicy (or highly seasoned) foods** that can aggravate heartburn.
- **Avoid going to bed on an empty stomach.**
- **Avoid over-eating before bed.** Eat heavier evening meals three hours before bed.
- **Avoid alcohol 4-6 hours before bedtime.** Although alcohol can have an immediate sleep-inducing effect (and some people think it helps them sleep better), for most, a few hours after drinking alcohol there is a rebound effect that can wake you up as it begins to leave the body. Alcohol can also negatively impact the quality of sleep.

Be informed

Eating several small, light, nutritious meals and drinking eight cups of fluid (water, herbal teas, broth or protein drinks) each day is generally agreed upon by health care providers to be the best way to begin eating following surgery.

The Importance of Hydration

The adult human body is mainly composed of water, 50-65% or more.

We hear a lot about the importance of drinking water and proper hydration these days. This is because our bodies depend on it! In general, lack of water will magnify or exaggerate any problems you may encounter after surgery. An ounce of prevention is so valuable; it's much easier to drink up than suffer the consequences.

Every system in the human body depends on water

Water is involved in almost every bodily function. It assists nearly every part and every system in the human body.

Water and surgery

Drinking extra water in the days before surgery prepares the body for the drying effects of surgery caused by anesthesia and other medications.[xviii] Drinking water after surgery facilitates healing, beginning with flushing and removing toxins from the system. Without sufficient hydration, the body cannot remove toxins or waste.

A soft drink is *not* the same as a glass of water. Soda pops contain unhealthy ingredients including phosphoric acid, high fructose corn syrup, caffeine, artificial colors, artificial flavors and artificial sweeteners, which are taxing to the liver which is already working harder than normal to flush surgical toxins.

Over 80% of the human body's daily requirement of water must be met by consuming fluids such as water, herbal teas or broths; the rest can be derived from food.

Drinking water:

- **Fends off dehydration** which can drain energy, affect mood and memory, make you tired, cause or worsen constipation and dry out eyes, nose and mouth
- **Transports essential nutrients and oxygen** to the body's cells and organs
- **Helps maintain proper muscle tone** and prevent painful muscle cramping, which can be triggered by dehydration and inactivity, both prior to and due to surgery

---

[xviii] Some post-surgery patients say that even with extra hydration their skin is exceptionally dry, itchy and in some cases peeling. This further illustrates how drying surgery, anesthesia and post-surgical medications can be. I have found that using coconut oil on dry areas, including my face, and taking liquid vitamin D3 and fish oil to have been helpful in combating severe dry skin.

- **Hydrates cells** so they can function properly and efficiently
- **Aids digestion** which can get out of whack after surgery
- **Removes waste.** Water assists the kidneys and liver in eliminating waste.
- **Protects and lubricates joints, organs and internal systems**
- **Connects brain synapses** so we can think
- **Regulates body temperature**

CONSIDER ADDING ELECTROLYTES TO A GLASS OF WATER

Electrolytes are needed to maintain proper fluid balance and to optimize energy levels so you can function at your best. A proper balance of fluids and electrolytes aids the body in recovery. Electrolytes regulate nerve and muscle function, hydration, blood pH, blood pressure and the rebuilding of damaged tissue. Trace Minerals Electrolyte Stamina Power Paks are an exceptional electrolyte. They contain more vitamin C, potassium and minerals and less sugar than other comparable brands. Trace Minerals can be found in health food stores, online through their website, TRACEMINERALS.COM, or on other websites such as AMAZON.COM.

Another healthy fluid high in electrolytes is coconut water. Coconut water is also high in potassium and magnesium and is rich in vitamins (especially B vitamins), minerals, trace elements (zinc, selenium, iodine, sulfur and manganese), amino acids, enzymes and antioxidants. Coconut water has anti-inflammatory and antimicrobial properties, aids rehydration and supports the immune system, digestion and kidney function. Unflavored, unsweetened coconut water also contains a moderate amount of natural sugar, but much less than fruit juices, sport drinks and soda pop. While natural sugar is better than artificial sugar, it's still sugar, so don't use coconut water exclusively to hydrate. Use in moderation with other healthy clear fluids.[xix]

[xix] Note: For those watching their sugar intake, be aware that some companies have added even more sugar to some coconut water products. Read the label.

Vitamins, Minerals and Herbs For Healing

In a perfect world the food we eat would give us all the nutrients—vitamins and minerals (also known as micro-nutrients)—our body needs to function optimally and heal. Unfortunately, this is probably not the case, at least for most people. It's certainly a much-debated, even controversial topic. Some question the necessity of vitamins or the added expense. Others argue that unless you breathe unpolluted air, have an unprocessed nutrient-dense diet with several servings of fresh fruits and vegetables a day, little stress, no digestive or absorption problems (or other health issues) and you have maximum energy and vitality, you may benefit from vitamin supplementation.

For me, I do everything I can to support healing which includes eating a nutrient-rich diet *and* supplementing with vitamins, minerals and herbs. Taking vitamins is something each individual will have to decide for themselves.

Are all vitamins the same?

In a word, no.

Okay, why?

Just like different food products contain different qualities of ingredients, so, too, do vitamins and supplements. Look for good quality vitamins that can be easily absorbed and utilized by the body. The best place to find quality vitamins is from a quality retailer with high standards, such as a health food store. One way to identify a good vitamin is to read the ingredient label on the back; see what fillers may have been added to it. Avoid products with unnecessary (and unhealthy) additives such as artificial color, sugar and hydrogenated oil.

The following two examples show the added ingredients found in a "good" vitamin and a "poor" vitamin. Both examples only show the fillers that have been added to a multi-vitamin and don't include the supplement facts or vitamin content.

This first example shows the added ingredients found in a good vitamin (Ultra Nutrient by PURE Encapsulations). Note: There is only one ingredient. This is an example of a vitamin completely free of unnecessary binders, fillers, artificial preservatives, colors and lubricants.

> other ingredients: vegetarian capsule (cellulose, water)

This second example is from a popular doctor-recommended brand. It contains numerous fillers, including three different artificial colors, hydrogenated palm oil, sugar and preservatives. Again, this is just the fillers and doesn't include the actual vitamin content which is listed separately.

> **Ingredients:** Calcium Carbonate, Potassium Chloride, Dibasic Calcium Phosphate, Magnesium Oxide, Ascorbic Acid (Vit. C), Microcrystalline Cellulose, dl-Alpha Tocopheryl Acetate (Vit. E), Pregelatinized Corn Starch, Modified Food Starch. **Contains < 2% of:** Acacia, Ascorbyl Palmitate, Beta-Carotene, BHT, Biotin, Boric Acid, Calcium Pantothenate, Calcium Stearate, Cholecalciferol (Vit. D$_3$), Chromium Picolinate, Citric Acid, Corn Starch, Crospovidone, Cupric Sulfate, Cyanocobalamin (Vit. B$_{12}$), FD&C Blue No. 2 Aluminum Lake, FD&C Red No. 40 Aluminum Lake, FD&C Yellow No. 6 Aluminum Lake, Folic Acid, Gelatin, Hydrogenated Palm Oil, Hypromellose, Lutein, Lycopene, Manganese Sulfate, Medium-Chain Triglycerides, Niacinamide, Nickelous Sulfate, Phytonadione (Vit. K), Polyethylene Glycol, Polyvinyl Alcohol, Potassium Iodide, Pyridoxine Hydrochloride (Vit. B$_6$), Riboflavin (Vit. B$_2$), Silicon Dioxide, Sodium Ascorbate, Sodium Benzoate, Sodium Borate, Sodium Citrate, Sodium Metavanadate, Sodium Molybdate, Sodium Selenate, Sorbic Acid, Sucrose, Talc, Thiamine Mononitrate (Vit. B$_1$), Titanium Dioxide, Tocopherols, Tribasic Calcium Phosphate, Vitamin A Acetate (Vit. A), Zinc Oxide. **May also contain < 2% of:** Maltodextrin, Sodium Aluminosilicate, Sunflower Oil.

The key to knowing what is in your vitamin is to take a minute and read both the supplement facts and the "other ingredients" listed on the label. (See page 204 for a list of some of my favorite brands.)

PRE- AND POST-OP VITAMIN, MINERAL AND HERB PROTOCOL

Preparing for and recovering from surgery are big jobs for the body and require a great deal of vitamins and minerals—again, much more than we probably usually consume on a regular daily basis. Recovery increases the demand for certain nutrients required for healing; nutrients that promote bone and tissue repair, reduce inflammation and more. Increasing vitamins and minerals during this time may be helpful for healing.

I have found a vitamin, mineral and herb routine before and after surgery to be valuable in my own health and recovery. Following reconstructive knee surgery, when I was on such a regimen, even though my surgeon didn't believe the vitamins, minerals and herbs I was taking were making any difference, he also could not account for the dramatically increased rate at which my healing progressed.

Unfortunately, most traditionally trained medical doctors aren't given formal education in this area. Any education or experience they have usually comes from their own research and discovery. Because some doctors lack knowledge and information, they often dismiss the benefits vitamins, minerals or herbs may have.

The good news is, today, more and more traditionally trained doctors are open to, or are incorporating, vitamins, minerals and herbs in their care, both to prepare patients for surgery and recover from surgery. If you have a belief system or experience that supports the use of vitamin, mineral and herb supplementation for health and healing, discuss it with your doctor. (See pages 199-201 for a sample vitamin, mineral and herb protocol for healing.)

I am fortunate to have a primary care physician who is exceptionally knowledgeable in this area. I believe the supplements, prescribed by my doctor, have made a difference for me, supporting and aiding my recovery on all levels—physically, mentally and emotionally.

PHYSICAL THERAPY

Surgeons can perform fantastical technical feats,
but it's a team effort and patients must to do their part.

■ ■ ■

Reducing pain and swelling and regaining any lost strength or mobility after surgery is an important part of a successful surgery (and recovery). To help you with this, your doctor will likely prescribe some physical therapy designed to make you feel better, help you heal and to get you back to your pre-surgery self.

Physical therapists are trained and licensed specialists. They work with you and your doctor to identify strengths, weaknesses and deficiencies in biomechanics. They use specialized tools, techniques and equipment and teach specific exercises and stretches to reduce swelling, provide pain relief, regain strength, coordination, balance, mobility and flexibility and restore well-being. Your physical therapist is there to support and assist you in getting back on your feet.

Depending on your procedure, you could be in physical therapy for anywhere from a few sessions to several months. Partner with your physical therapist. Communicate both pain and progress to them so they can choose the best tools for you and make adjustments along the way. Follow through with home exercises and stretching and attend all appointments for the best results.

For me, the more I've communicated with my physical therapist, the more I've gotten out of the experience. Share your post-surgery goals with them. Tell them what you love to do and want to get back to doing. If you're visual, like me, create an inspiration board or hang images of yourself around your house doing what you love, so you can see yourself healthy and happy. You can see some of my inspirations on page 94.

PHYSICAL THERAPY TOOLS MAY INCLUDE:

- **Heat**. Heat is useful in warming up an area before working it.
- **Ice**. Ice is useful in cooling down muscles. The alternative use of heat and ice in a physical therapy setting can additionally stimulate blood flow and decrease swelling.
- **Ultrasound**. Ultrasound uses high frequency sound waves to penetrate and stimulate deep tissues. Ultrasound can be valuable in the healing and regenerating process. It gets tissue molecules moving, increases blood flow to tissues and draws blood containing oxygen and nutrients to an injured area.

Ultrasound following surgery can also be used to warm up an area prior to physical therapy sessions and to reduce swelling by dissipating pooled fluids from a surgical site. It can also help keep an incision and the surrounding tissue pliable by breaking down scar tissue.

- **Electrical stimulation** (also referred to as TENS, transcutaneous electrical neural stimulation). TENS is a therapy that passes an electrical current to an affected area or muscle group altering nerve conduction. This causes increased blood flow to the tissue and makes the muscle contract, which can help strengthen it and prevent atrophy. The low voltage electrical impulses of TENS can also disrupt pain cycles. Depending on the frequency the machine is set at, it may stimulate the body to release endorphins, the body's natural painkillers. Patients often experience diminished pain following electrical stimulation treatments. TENS isn't a curative measure, but has been shown to be effective in treating acute pain.

- **Stretching tight muscles and joints**. Stretching can assist in regaining range-of-motion and flexibility. Stretching surgical areas after surgery can also assist in breaking down scar tissue that traditionally forms following surgery or an injury.

- **Localized manual therapy**. This is a clinical, hands-on approach used by physical therapists to treat musculoskeletal pain and disability, increase range of motion, reduce or eliminate excessive inflammation, facilitate movement and improve function. Manual therapy commonly includes kneading and manipulation of muscles and joints to decrease pain.

- **Strengthening exercises**. Exercises, exercise machines and free weights may be used to help improve muscle strength, function and endurance. Depending on your procedure, some restrictions may exist, so follow your physical therapist's directions carefully.

Play date with daughter-in-law & grandson

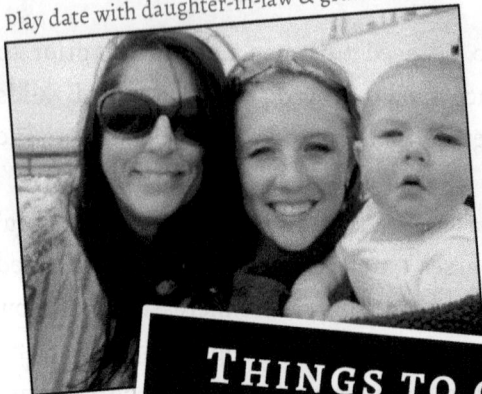

Ennis, Montana with Bert

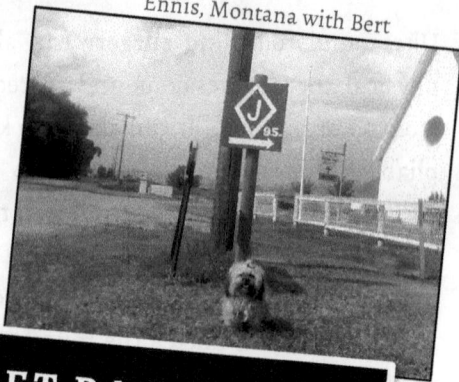

THINGS TO GET BACK TO ...

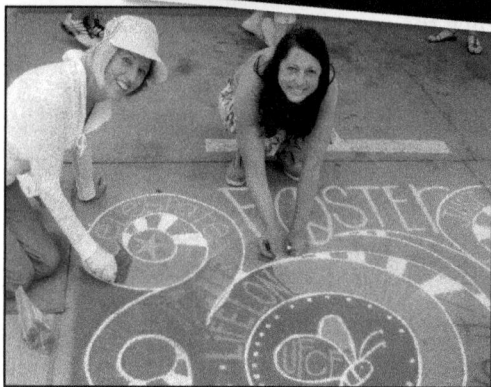

Chalk Art Festival for Utah Foster Care with Mom

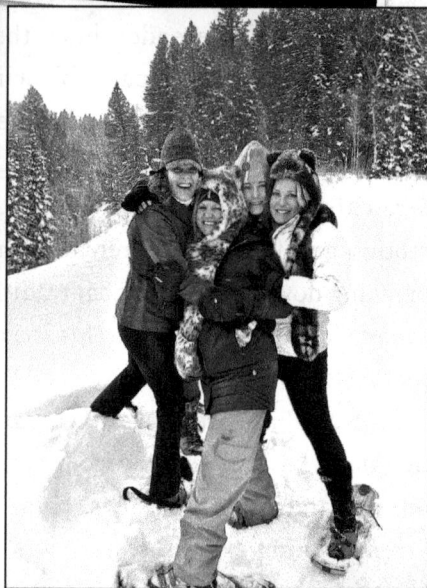

Snowshoeing with friends, Solitude, Utah

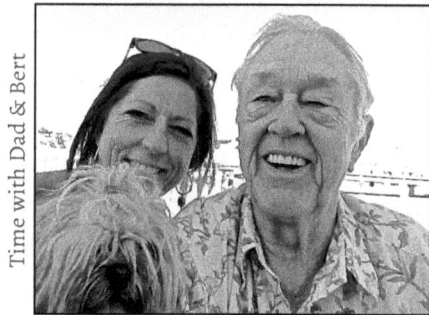

Time with Dad & Bert

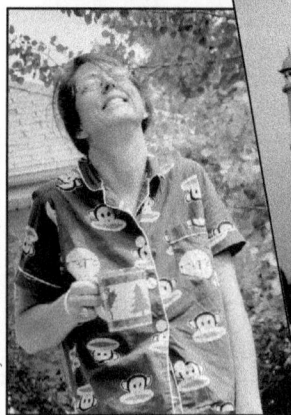

Photo by Stacie Isabella Turk/Ribbonhead ©

Home, Salt Lake City, Utah

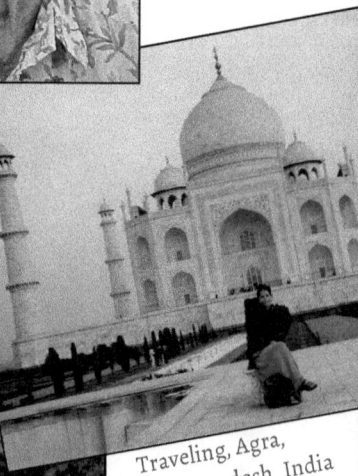

Traveling, Agra,
Uttar Pradesh, India

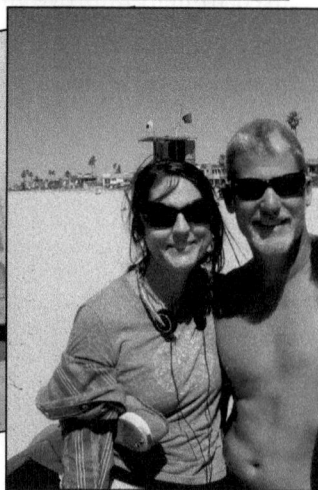

The Wedge,
Newport Beach, California

94

THE BENEFITS OF EXERCISE

. . .

Exercise is an integral part of wellness and plays a vital role in healing. Maintaining an exercise routine (if possible) before surgery can be valuable for strengthening, stability and a quicker comeback following surgery—the more you can do for yourself physically before surgery, the better off you will be after. Exercise after surgery, when permitted, can help with healing on all levels, physically, mentally and emotionally. Check with your doctor for any restrictions before starting a pre- or post-operative exercise routine.

THE BENEFITS OF REGULAR EXERCISE BEFORE AND AFTER SURGERY INCLUDE:

- **Speeding wound healing**. Wounds tend to heal more quickly in individuals who exercise regularly.
- **Strength**. Strength generated by exercise prior to surgery can help with balance and stability after surgery. A strong core and strong lower body muscles will keep you more solid on your feet, aid in getting in and out of a chair or bed more easily and help maintain balance when moving or reaching for something.
- **Better/increased circulation**. Increased circulation delivers oxygen and nutrients to tissues and helps the cardiovascular system work better. Increased blood flow also helps sweep debris away from the injury site and brings in macrophages[xx] to clean up the rest. It also keeps organs and other bodily systems functioning regularly, which can, in turn, contribute to a quicker recovery. Exercise can also be helpful in relieving constipation.
- **Prevention of muscle atrophy**. Atrophy begins the minute we stop moving.
- **Keeping injured joints or joints around an injury mobile**. Exercise can help prevent the body from creating excessive scar tissue, which can cause an injured joint to become stiff.
- **Improved mood**. Physical activity encourages the production and release of endorphins, which can give your spirits a boost and aid in pain control. Exercise, even moderate light exercise, can also be a great way to ease anxiety and tension. Rhythmic breathing from exercise can have a calming effect on the mind.
- **Getting a better night's rest**. Regular exercise can improve sleep by helping you fall asleep and get a deeper, more restful, healing night's sleep.

[xx] Macrophages are cells highly specialized in removing dead cells and other cellular debris.

- **A boost in energy.** Regular physical activity strengthens muscles and improves endurance, which can translate to more energy and reduced fatigue.
- **Normalizing (and regulating) cortisol levels[xxi], insulin, blood glucose, growth hormones and thyroid hormones.** Cortisol is a hormone the body produces and releases in response to stress, including trauma or surgery. While cortisol helps maintain the body's systems when under stress, prolonged, elevated cortisol in the system can have a negative effect.[17,18,19]

[xxi] A bit about cortisol and its role in stress, surgery and healing. Studies reveal that physically and emotionally stressful times (especially long periods of ongoing stress) can weaken the body's immune system, making it more susceptible to infection and other illnesses. Thankfully, the body has built-in support mechanisms—the adrenal glands—to help. The adrenal glands produce a variety of valuable healing hormones to support the body and brain through stressful times such as surgery. Many are familiar with the primary hormone produced by the adrenal glands, adrenaline.

Adrenaline is the body's first line of support and is released in emergency situations—when we are scared or fighting for survival. Among other jobs in the body, adrenaline is responsible for the "fight or flight" response. In an emergency, adrenaline is the first responding hormone that gives the body super-human strength needed to survive—it's a good thing. The next responding adrenal hormone is cortisol which provides long-term support. Cortisol supports healing, energy levels and helps the body through stressful physical and emotional periods. (In addition to adrenaline and cortisol, the adrenal glands produce other important hormones, the most prominent and important being DHEA and aldosterone, which mediate our long-term response to stress.)

However, if cortisol stays elevated in the body for long periods of time, such as during a long recovery or extended period of stress, the adrenal glands can become exhausted and burn out (also called adrenal fatigue). This can leave the body and mind depleted and vulnerable to a host of other symptoms ranging from exhaustion to emotional sensitivity to lowered immunity and poor wound healing. These are not caused by cortisol, but can be effects of ongoing, long-term stress.

While some doctors today recognize adrenal fatigue, much of the mainstream medical collective only acknowledge complete adrenal failure, also called adrenal insufficiency or Addison's disease. To deal with the symptoms of adrenal fatigue that mimic depression (exhaustion, apathy, mood swings, low energy, low stamina and loss of interest in sex), many doctors prescribe anti-depressants. Adrenal fatigue can also weaken resistance to infection, cause low blood pressure, low blood sugar and the need for excessive amounts of sleep. Unfortunately, to counter these symptoms, people often consume sugar, carbohydrates and caffeine to give them energy and make them temporarily feel better, but this just further compounds the problem.

Acknowledging and managing stress and eating a nutrient-rich diet can help keep cortisol levels in check and the adrenal glands healthy so they can support your recovery.

THERE ARE MANY WAYS TO STIMULATE CIRCULATION AND IMPROVE CONDITIONING

Once cleared by your surgeon and physical therapist, you can begin or resume an exercise program. Ease into any workout schedule. Start with gentle exercises or classes, such as light massage, soothing yoga or walking. As your strength and endurance improve, include more strenuous exercises. There are lots of ways to move the body and get the blood flowing; the following are just a few.

- **Walking or jogging.** Inside or outside, even for 10-15 minutes, increases the circulation of blood and oxygen. Done outside, fresh air and sunshine also stimulate the pineal gland, which contributes to an overall sense of well-being. I am lucky to live in Salt Lake City where there are great parks within walking distance of my home and easy hikes just a five to ten minute drive. For me, getting fresh air and sun can make a big difference in how I feel. Being in nature also helps clear my mind. When I'm outside and moving I often get bursts of clarity and insight. For that reason, I carry a pen and paper (along with some water). I like to plug in my headphones and turn up the music too. You may sometimes recognize me by my disco walking and the occasional singing out loud. Might look silly (and sound off key), but I'm having fun!
- **Weights**. Resistance training using free-weights or machines builds strength.
- **Yoga**. Yoga classes, techniques and teachers vary greatly. There are many styles of yoga ranging from very relaxing to extremely aerobic and competitive. Find the style and teacher that are the right fit and the right pace for you. A good place to start may be with a gentle hatha or restorative yoga class. If you're not sure which class is right for you, ask at a studio and talk to some teachers. Find a teacher who is willing to work with you on your recovery.
- **Pool exercises**. Check your YMCA or local aquatic center for water classes that are energizing and low impact, or, keep it simple and take a walk in the pool. My friend Jane and I like to water walk. I like it because we get to spend time together walking, talking and laughing and since water is twelve times more resistant than air, with every low-impact step we also get a workout. Remember, getting in a pool is only advised once an incision is closed and any scab has fallen off.
- **Biking**. Biking can be a great activity whether it's inside on a stationary bike or outside, around the park. Got to love a ride in the park (with a helmet, of course).
- **Stationary equipment**. There is a wide variety of stationary equipment available that can be good sources of exercise; treadmills, Stairmasters, elliptical and rowing machines are usually available at most gyms. Start out slow and build from there.

GET A WORKOUT PARTNER

For me, having a workout partner helps make me more accountable and less likely to flake on a workout. A workout partner also can make it fun! Never underestimate the value of a friend or partner to get you going or help keep you going.

CAN I HAVE SEX NOW?

You are not the first person to ask this question.

■ ■ ■

Sex after surgery is a common question, yet one patients are often too embarrassed to ask. Ask. Doctors have answered this question many times.

GENERAL GUIDELINES FOR SEX AFTER SURGERY

You should be able to have sex when you are able to return to work and to full physical activity. For example, when your doctor says, "You should be able to return to your normal activities in [INSERT # HERE] days/weeks," this is a good indicator that you may resume your sex life as well.

After some surgeries, such as open-heart surgery, you may feel fully recovered but be at risk if you exert yourself too much. If your doctor cautions you against strenuous activity such as running, brisk aerobic activity or shoveling snow, you should consider this a caution regarding having sex, too.

Surgeries that affect the reproductive organs, such as inguinal hernia repairs, hysterectomies, prostate surgeries or any surgery directly involving the penis or vagina may require additional healing time prior to engaging in sex as well.

Listen to your body and let pain be your guide. If you experience pain during intercourse, this is your body telling you it's not ready and needs more time to heal. If your sex drive has dramatically changed following surgery, or is just plain off, it may be off for a reason. It may be your body's way of telling you it needs more rest or it could be that your hormones are off. If your sex drive stays off longer than you've been advised it might, ask your doctor about it and see if there is a medical reason for the change that needs to be addressed.

FACTORS THAT CAN IMPACT FEELINGS OR DESIRE FOR SEX AFTER SURGERY:

- **Medication side effects** that zap sexual potency and desire, or cause impotence
- **Lack of energy** due to your system using it all to heal
- **Fear** about re-injuring a newly repaired area
- **Depression**
- **Hormone imbalances** caused by the stress of surgery on the body

TALK ABOUT IT

Communication between you and your doctor and communication between you and your partner are key. With lots going on physically, mentally and emotionally following surgery, it is especially important to communicate with your partner about where you are physically and how you are feeling emotionally.

Sometimes, in spite of all our best efforts, we are just off in this area for no explainable reason. If this is the case for you, try not to judge yourself. Instead, be patient. Give yourself and your body—your whole body, not just your surgery site—more time to rest and heal. I have spent time myself in this dull-feeling void area. What I can share is that sometimes the answer is simply to communicate how you're feeling to the best of your ability and then do nothing. When I've let go of trying to make something (a situation, for example) be what I want it to be and simply allowed it to be what it was, a little time allowed the situation to naturally resolve itself.

QUESTIONS YOU AND YOUR PARTNER MAY WANT TO DISCUSS BEFORE HAVING SEX FOLLOWING SURGERY:

- Is it safe? Any chance sex could cause harm to the surgical repair or site?
- Do you "feel" like having sex?
- Do you have the physical energy at this time?
- Do you need to avoid putting pressure on a certain area, such as an incision line?
- Are some positions more comfortable—or uncomfortable—than others?
- Do any of the medications you are taking impact the effectiveness of birth control pills? Do you need to use a back-up birth control method? (For example, some antibiotics cause the birth control pill to be ineffective. I know of doctors who have failed to mention this to patients who then have gotten pregnant.)
- Is there any physical reason to avoid getting pregnant following surgery? Because of the surgery, are you now taking any medications that could negatively impact a pregnancy, making conception contraindicated or inadvisable?
- Will you need to take any special measures? Some surgeries, such as vaginal surgeries, may cause dryness and make a lubricant necessary. Other surgeries, such as prostate surgery, may make an erection difficult to obtain or maintain.

WEIGHT LOSS AND WEIGHT GAIN AFTER SURGERY

...

Following surgery (or other major trauma or illness), many people experience mild to significant weight loss or weight gain. This is fairly common.

WEIGHT LOSS

Lack of appetite after surgery is normal and typically passes in a few days. Some people have extra padding that the body can shed following surgery and some people lose weight they need to retain. Either way, eating is important. The body needs the energy and nutrients from food to heal; stress and trauma to the body use up more energy and nutrients than normal.

While pain and assorted medications can cause a lack of appetite, not eating enough healthy foods following surgery can slow healing, cause constipation or delay the closure of an incision. Physical pain and some medications can also cause nausea and vomiting.

If you are feeling nauseated for any reason, a little food in your stomach (a simple scrambled egg, crackers or half a banana, for example) may help. If symptoms last for more than a day or two, bring it to the attention of your doctor. It's possible your doctor may prescribe some anti-nausea medication to alleviate symptoms.

WEIGHT GAIN

Conversely, some patients may experience weight gain following surgery. This can be a side effect of some medications, due to inactivity or a combination of both. As you heal and get back to your normal routine, any weight gain should also correct itself. If the weight you've gained feels particularly abnormal for you and your body, talk about it with your doctor.

THE POST-OP BLUES

• • •

Depending on the patient and the surgical procedure, there are several emotions—high and low—that a patient may experience before and after surgery. Prior to surgery, patients may be anxious about being prepared and about the surgery itself. Following surgery, even if patients are in pain, they may feel relieved—even euphoric—knowing that the worst is behind them and they survived. Patients can feel these emotions over a week, a day, or all at the same time. Feelings that occur all at once or in rapid succession can be confusing and overwhelming.

After the relief of surviving surgery wears off, and the pain and discomfort that can be associated with healing and recovery set in, so, too, can the post-op blues.

IT'S NORMAL. YOU ARE NORMAL!

Following surgery, it's normal to feel tired, irritable, run-down or lacking in energy. Some may also experience emotional letdown—the post-op blues—which they aren't prepared for that can amplify tired, irritable, run-down feelings. Feelings and emotions may be less tangible, but they are no less real.

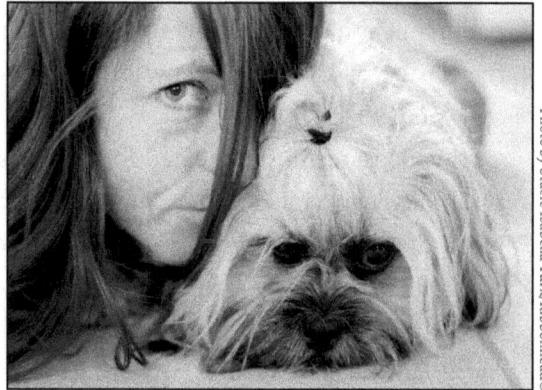

Photo by Stacie Isabella Turk/Ribbonhead©

THE BLUES CAN BE TRIGGERED OR CAUSED BY:

- **Mental and emotional stress** following the diagnosis of an illness or injury
- **Fear, worry, anxiety**
- **Physical stress** including the traumatic physical impact of surgery on the body
- **Pain**, especially ongoing pain
- **Mood altering medications** that can interfere with brain neurochemistry
- **Anesthesia**
- **Financial concerns**: bills, loss of work
- **Poor diet** and eating habits
- **Disrupted sleep**, lack of rest, exhaustion
- **Confinement** to bed
- **Inactivity** for extended periods
- **Lack of exercise**
- **Lack of sunshine**, natural light, fresh air
- **Lifestyle changes**
- **Frustration** from feeling like healing isn't progressing or is taking forever
- **Unrealistic expectations** regarding the length of time healing can take
- **Fear you won't ever feel "normal"**

DEPRESSION AND SURGERY

If the post-op blues hang around too long they can turn into depression. Depression does not affect everyone the same way. For some, it can be triggered by a diagnosis that leads to surgery, by a lengthy healing and recovery process or, it may be triggered by some prescribed medications. Individuals with a personal or family history of depression may also be more likely to develop depression during stress-filled times, such as preparing for and going through surgery. Acknowledged, depression can be managed along the way. Ignored, depression can be serious and lead to difficulty with day-to-day life, impaired decision-making and slower healing and recovery times. Being aware of depression is important so that if it does occur, it can be identified and treated.

SIGNS AND SYMPTOMS OF DEPRESSION INCLUDE:

- **Eating significantly more or less** than normal
- **Insomnia** *or* **sleeping significantly more** than normal
- **Fatigue** or malaise
- **Lack of enthusiasm**
- **Loss of interest in activities**

- **Difficulty making simple decisions**
- **Excessive sadness**
- **More sensitive** or emotional than normal
- **Irritability** or angry outbursts
- **Feelings of hopelessness** and despair
- **Suicidal thoughts** (seek immediate help)

Since having surgery can also disrupt sleep, appetite and energy, it can sometimes be difficult to distinguish "normal" symptoms associated with undergoing surgery from those of depression. Simply be aware of how you are feeling and whether or not the feelings subside and get better over time. Ongoing physical and emotional symptoms may indicate a problem.

If you experience symptoms that don't seem to be improving following surgery, it may be time to ask for help. While medical intervention may be necessary in treating depression, there are also things you can do to support yourself.

BE AWARE

Whether it's preparing for surgery or recovering from surgery, acknowledge what's going on: You have a lot on your plate. In an interview, author Wayne Dyer put it simply,

"When (you) become aware, (you) can become pro-active."

Once you're aware of what's going on, you can take steps to lighten your load and let go of things that may be weighing heavy on your mind. To accomplish this, consciously put some mental and emotional support into place and use it.

WHAT DO MENTAL AND EMOTIONAL SUPPORT LOOK LIKE?

Pages 11-16 described creating a team to support your physical well-being in practical and physical ways. However, it's important to also have support for your mental and emotional well-being. This includes people you can share your feelings with, who can listen and provide feedback, a different perspective and encouragement through a possibly scary time.

MENTAL AND EMOTIONAL SUPPORT TEAM IDEAS:

- **Family and friends**
- **Medical team members**: surgeon, doctor, physical therapist. Share with them.
- **Licensed counselor, therapist or life coach**
- **Religious leader or spiritual teacher**
- **Church, congregation or spiritual community**
- **Yoga instructor, personal trainer or other instructor** and classmates
- **Athletic coach, teammates** or other injured recovering players
- **Hospital support groups**. Some hospitals have support groups for surgery, pain management, depression, trauma and more.
- **Online support groups**. Note: Be careful to avoid groups that are overly negative or harsh, which can be counterproductive and cause more stress and anxiety.

On various occasions, my mental and emotional support team has included family members, friends, my yoga instructor, counselor, spiritual advisor and spiritual community.

Having been through a challenging and lengthy recovery from my head injury, I found myself particularly scared and anxious when I was faced with undergoing back surgery, even though it was considered safe and "minor," comparatively. But, my feelings were my feelings and I was overwhelmed. Additionally, in the months prior to surgery, I was in a significant amount of pain that caused me to be on fairly strong pain management medications, which I believe compounded my anxious feelings. In any event, my surgery was successful and I walked out of the surgical center in very little pain compared to when I checked in. I was grateful for the support I had in place; they picked me up when I was down and helped carry me through.

USE THE RESOURCES YOU PUT INTO PLACE

Rather than staying stuck, feeling lost or alone, prepare the best you can and then use the resources you've identified and put into place; set up a regular self-care routine.

It's worth repeating:

A diagnosis that requires surgery
may trigger a wide range of feelings and emotions.
Anxiety, fear, frustration, hopelessness, helplessness, despair and depression
are common feelings you may experience.

EVERYONE'S EXPERIENCE IS DIFFERENT

I've battled the post-op blues. Following open-heart surgery when I was 22 years old, I remember feeling grateful the congenital defect in my heart had been successfully repaired and that I didn't wake up with a pacemaker (which was a possibility). However, 12 days later, after I was discharged from the hospital, the fear, pain, stiffness and general discomfort from the physical trauma of having my chest cracked open really settled in. It hurt and I was nervous about moving around. On some level, I thought my chest might split back open. Emotionally I was afraid that because I had a scar down the center of my chest I was somehow less attractive. Healing both physically and emotionally took many months.

That was my experience, but not everyone's experience is the same. Twenty-four years later, my friend's 17-year-old daughter had open-heart surgery. While our procedures had similarities, our post-op experiences were different; she bounced back faster than I did. She felt great and was pain-free in four weeks. Her posture was gorgeous and she proudly wore her scar like an honor badge.

I love this contrast. While both experiences were real and true, it's also true that everyone's experiences and recoveries are different. It was inspiring to me to hear her story and see how she was thriving.

Even though healing can sometimes be slow going, it gets better; *healing occurs naturally, all the time, whether we're aware of it or not.*

The good news is: The post-op blues don't last forever.

EASING SYMPTOMS OF THE POST-OP BLUES AND DEPRESSION

The following are some ideas for easing symptoms of the post-op blues and depression. Use what resonates for you and discard the rest.

HARNESSING THE POWER OF YOUR MIND AND EMOTIONS

Harnessing the power of our mind and emotions means not letting fear or negativity define us or bog us down. When the body is under duress, the mind and our emotions are also impacted—it's all connected. In short, pay attention to your emotions.

Emotions are how the body expresses itself;
they are the connection between the mind and the body.

Acknowledge emotions and then try to understand why you are having them. For some, emotions and feelings may not be comfortable, but they are normal. As you heal and the physical resolves, so, too, will the emotional. Know that if you are struggling, you won't feel like this forever, even if that's how it feels in the moment. Feelings of frustration are understandable but not productive; they only waste energy. Try not to judge. Instead, accept where you are—on the road to recovery—and move forward one step at a time.

MONITOR YOUR THOUGHTS

If you experience troubling or upsetting feelings, acknowledge them, but don't continue to ruminate on them. Your mental and emotional health can and do affect your physical health. Cutting edge neuroscience studies confirm that continued replication—continual thinking—of negative or self-critical thoughts can literally change the brain's chemistry. The altered chemistry then loops back around and serves to continue negative thinking and feeling through a depressed emotional state. This eventually causes a groove in our thinking (like a scratch on a record) and the negative feedback loop continues.[20] Luckily, the same is true of a positive feedback loop, only rather than depressed emotional states, the positive feedback loop causes light, hopeful, enthusiastic states.

"As he thinks, so he is: As he continues to think, so he remains."
James Allen

MRIs have shown that when people start to think happy thoughts, a surge of blood flows into brain regions associated with happiness—widening their positive neural pathways and making it easier and more automatic for them to think better, calmer thoughts. If you keep focusing on those happy thoughts, over time it will become easier and easier to think more positively.[21] It is from this state that the realm of possibility can be accessed.

If you need help getting started, try the 100 Happy Days challenge at 100HAPPYDAYS.COM. My friends and I have done it and it was easy, fun and generated many smiles.

THE MIND-BODY CONNECTION

In the spring of 2013, because of my volunteer affiliation at the George E. Wahlen Veterans Affairs Medical Center in Salt Lake City, I was able to attend a talk by Tracy Gaudet, M.D. Dr. Gaudet is the Director of the Department of Veterans Affairs Office of Patient Centered Care and Cultural Transformation. I was thrilled to hear her speak about patient-centered care, acknowledging the mind-body connection and discussing the power of our words and thoughts. Dr. Gaudet was very clear:

"The power of words is huge!"

Beginning in the 1980s I read books that introduced me to various perspectives and possibilities regarding healing and the mind. Author Norman Cousins, *Anatomy of An Illness*, did research on the mind and human emotions, which he believed were the key to our success in fighting illness.[22] *Love, Medicine & Miracles* by Bernie Siegel, M.D., is about the power of love to heal, which was based on his personal and professional experiences with patient after patient.

"Unconditional love is the most powerful stimulant of the immune system.
The truth is: love heals.
Miracles happen to patients every day—
patients who have the courage to love, those who have the courage to
work with their doctors to participate in and influence their own recovery."[23]

At the time, Dr. Siegel's words hit home for me on a personal level as I explored partnership with my own doctors and prepared for open-heart surgery.

New York Times best-selling authors Deepak Chopra, M.D., Andrew Weil, M.D. and Wayne Dyer, Ph.D. have been writing books and lecturing for decades about their experiences with patients and the mind-body connection and the importance of paying attention to our thoughts.

Stem cell biologist and best-selling author of *The Biology of Belief,* Bruce Lipton, Ph.D., takes a scientific approach, studying and sharing about the connection between feelings and cellular biology. How when we feel love, joy and warmth our body releases chemicals—dopamine, oxytocin, vasopressin and growth hormone—which cause cells to grow exuberantly well (following surgery this translates to healing). He also shares about the experience of fear and how it releases an entirely different set of chemicals. Fear causes the body to release stress hormones and inflammatory agents into the system. When the body does this, the cells stop growing in an effort to conserve energy. "Don't grow if you have to fight or run away (from danger). Stop growing (healing) and use that energy for escape." Now, multiply this by 50 trillion. Yup, the human body is comprised of more than 50 trillion cells, all responding to emotional signals (joy, love, fear) we send 24 hours a day.[24]

Food for thought... What are you focusing on or giving your attention too?

> *As you become more and more aware of the interconnectedness*
> *of the body, mind, spirit and emotions within your own being,*
> *you will also become aware of how each impacts the other.*

LOOK AT POSSIBLE MEDICATION SIDE EFFECTS

Are you experiencing any medication side effects? As mentioned on page 64, some medications, especially opiate-based pain medications, can cause or deepen depression. Go over all your medications with your doctor to see if any of them could be causing or compounding blue feelings.

GIVE YOURSELF PERMISSION TO BE WHERE YOU ARE—JUST BE

If you're feeling overwhelmed or stuck, give yourself permission to just be where you are, feeling how you're feeling. Give yourself permission to stop and regroup. I've done this countless times. For me, I hit the pause button. Sometimes the pause is brief and sometimes it lasts until the next day, it just depends. For me it can look like retreating to a warm bath or sometimes I just go back to bed—it's amazing the benefits one can reap from a timeout or nap. I also give myself permission to not get everything done; permission to say 'yes' and let others help me; permission to say 'no' if I am tired; and permission to not be perfect. I give myself permission to simply be where I am, which sometimes is "up" and, admittedly, sometimes is "down." Take a minute and,

Reflect on all you've been through and
acknowledge how far you've come!

Do your best to focus on the progress you have made and are continuing to make. Celebrate the small improvements—they add up. Small progress is still progress!

TALK IT OUT

Given that preparing for and recovering from surgery can be stressful, sometimes talking it through with a professional counselor or therapist can help lift burdens and fears; keeping feelings inside can make you feel worse. Unaddressed feelings can also get distorted and blown out of proportion. Sometimes saying something out loud allows us to hear it differently. When I have felt overwhelmed prior to or after surgery, I've successfully used a licensed therapist as a sounding board. What I learned is that while feelings are valid, the stories we make up about them may not be valid or true. Sometimes, someone outside a situation can help us sort through what's real and true in a situation that may feel bleak. Sharing feelings with a trusted friend or family member can also be helpful. It's okay to let loved ones know when something is bothering you.

CHANGE YOUR MIND

"When you change the way you look at things,
the things you look at change."
Wayne Dyer

If you're feeling stuck, make a decision to take a step forward, even if it's a small one. Take a deep breath. Go outside and feel the warmth of the sun. Do something different. Switch up your routine.

USE GRATITUDE

When I have felt frustrated or like my recovery has stalled, I've used gratitude to shift my focus and energy. On numerous occasions, at bedtime, I would take a minute and write down everything I was grateful for that day: more energy or mobility, less pain, a friendly smile, a flower I noticed blooming outside the window—anything that gave me peace or joy, big or small. What I found was that focusing a little time and attention on the things that went right and felt good caused them to multiply. Energy goes where attention flows.

WRITE IT DOWN AND FORGET ABOUT IT

When I'm feeling really anxious and cannot think my way through a problem, I write down what is bothering or gnawing away at me on a small piece of paper. If there's something I can do about it in the moment, I do it. If not, I fold the paper up, tuck it away and forget about it. I write my greatest problems and fears down and release them. What I have found over and over again is that everything I've ever written down has gotten solved and resolved, but not because I did anything, but rather because I did nothing—I was willing to simply write it down and let it go.

I like how author and teacher Byron Katie puts it,

"It's not the problem that causes our suffering;
it's our thinking about the problem."

When I feel stuck I also use *The Serenity Prayer*:

"Grant me the serenity to
Accept the things I cannot change;
The courage to change the things that I can;
And the wisdom to know the difference!"[25]

HUG YOUR PET

One day, when I was inconsolable from back pain, I called a friend for support. Knowing I was alone and scared, she told me to pick up my dog and feel for his heartbeat. I did what she said, but couldn't hear or feel a thing because I was crying. It took a few minutes, but the act of listening to my friend's calm voice and feeling for my dog's heartbeat forced me to slow my breathing and become single focused and present. It was then that I felt his little heart beat. In that moment I was still. My breathing was slow and steady and my concentration fully focused outside of myself and my pain. Relaxing to feel for my dog's heartbeat reduced my pain. Look for the heartbeat—your own or that of a beloved pet. Thank you Stacie.

SUNSHINE AND FRESH AIR

Both sunshine and fresh air are known to help bust the blues. They can assist in re-regulating circadian (sleep) rhythms and alleviate symptoms of depression. Vitamin D3, also known as the sunshine vitamin, has been shown to protect against insomnia and depression. The two primary ways to get vitamin D3 are from direct sunlight or supplementation. If you live in North America, due to the angle of the sun, especially in the winter months, it's not possible to get enough UV light for the skin to make vitamin D3, so supplementation may be the best way to make sure you're getting enough. Your doctor can order a blood test to check levels if you think you may be low on vitamin D3. In the meantime, the first step: Open the door and step outside.

EXERCISE (AND DANCING)

Light exercise (including dancing), when permitted, can be a great mood stabilizer. When you exercise, your body releases hormones called endorphins, which trigger positive feelings and pleasure in the body. Endorphins also act as natural painkillers. Regular exercise has been proven to reduce stress, ward off anxiety and depression and improve sleep. (See pages 95-98 for more on the benefits of exercise and some exercise ideas.) For me, sometimes a spontaneous mini dance party in my living room does just the trick.[xxii]

PUT ON SOME GOOD MUSIC

When I'm feeling stuck or blue, music can help get me moving and help shift me out of the doldrums. A couple of my current favorites are, *"Happy"* by Pharrell Williams, *"I'm Alive"* by the Electric Light Orchestra and *"All You Need is Love"* by the Beatles. Or try starting your day with the *"Peter Gunn Theme"* from the 60s, that always makes me smile.

GOOD FOOD = GOOD MOOD

A healthy diet and proper hydration can help fight depression! (Refer to pages 77-88 for information on a nutrient-rich diet rich that supports healing, physically and emotionally.)

GET MORE SLEEP—TAKE A NAP

The critical nature of sleep and rest was covered on pages 72-76. Sleep is required for healing and the release of healing growth hormones. Poor sleep or lack of sleep can cause myriad problems including fatigue, loss of motivation and depression. Being diligent about getting enough proper, restorative rest is super crucial following surgery. Go to bed earlier; add naps. It's not forever, but it's what your body may need right now.

[xxii] Having said that, if I'm being honest, when I'm feeling blue, turning on the music or getting out of the house can be a hard first step. This is where I have found friends to be helpful. Sometimes we need a little coaxing and encouragement. I have been grateful for emails, texts and calls from friends wanting to listen and help.

MASSAGE THERAPY AND BODYWORK

Massage therapy and bodywork are wonderful tools for healing and easing the blues. Check with your doctor to make sure receiving bodywork is safe for you and then tap into your network and get a referral for a good licensed massage therapist. (See pages 69-70 about the benefits of massage therapy and pages 192-194 for more on massage therapy and bodywork techniques).

NEWS FAST

For some (like me), eliminating news can be helpful, especially if I'm feeling vulnerable or tired. Remember the example from Dr. Lipton on pages 108? Positive feelings cause feel-good chemicals to be released into the body. Fear and anxiety, from bad news for example, can cause the release of stress hormones and inflammatory agents. Turn off the news (television and radio) and toss the newspaper. See if you notice a difference in how you feel.

CALM YOUR MIND (AND BODY)—THE POWER OF VISUALIZATION

Calm feelings help activate healing processes within the body. When life feels like it's spinning out of control, calming the mind can help restore balance. It's also from a calm still place that we can change the way we perceive and react to a situation.

CALMING THE MIND SUCCESSFULLY HELPS:

- **Shorten hospital stays**
- **Enhance sleep**
- **Decrease pain and the need for post-surgical pain medication**—some pain medications have been known to worsen negative feelings or depression.
- **Decrease some side effects of medical procedures and medicines**
- **Decrease anxiety, frustration, worry and fear**
- **Decrease feelings of loneliness, hopelessness, helplessness and depression**
- **Increase overall sense of well-being**
- **Strengthen the immune system and enhance the body's natural ability to heal**
- **Reduce recovery time**

One powerful method to calm the mind and body is visualization. Visualization has been documented to be powerful before, during and after surgery for anxiety, pain management and healing, among other benefits. Hospitals across the U.S., including Brigham and Women's Hospital in Boston, recommend visualization.

One program, *Prepare for Surgery, Heal Faster: A Guide of Mind Body Techniques* by Peggy Huddleston, shows how to use mind-body techniques to reduce anxiety, use 23-50% less pain medication and heal faster.[26] Lawrence Cohn, M.D., cardiac surgeon and Professor of Cardiac Surgery at Harvard Medical School, says that:

> *Anything a patient does to relieve anxiety will generate a better surgical outcome and contribute to a successful surgery.*

Sometimes, a patient is so anxious that it causes them to have negative interactions with doctors, nurses and aids trying to help and care for them. One heart-surgery patient of Dr. Cohn's used *Prepare for Surgery, Heal Faster* before, during and after her surgery and said it helped bring her off the ceiling; that she really felt she did better with the program: more comfortable, more relaxed and more in control.[27]

There are many visualization techniques and exercises. The one you resonate with is the one that you will be the most successful using. (See examples on page 198.)

SHARE WITH YOUR DOCTOR

The time before and after surgery can be stressful. It's important to share both physical and emotional symptoms with your doctor. This includes negative, dark or depressed feelings you may be having, even if you're not used to sharing or totally comfortable doing so. Some people don't like to label or discuss negative feelings, but it is important to acknowledge them because,

> *Ongoing negative feelings that don't resolve as you heal can compromise your health and impede your recovery.*[28,29]

Ongoing anxiety, despair, hopelessness or depression that doesn't improve with time can be treatable through a variety of traditional and non-traditional methods.

POST-SURGICAL DOCTOR FOLLOW UP

. . .

See your doctor for post-surgical follow-up visits as directed. This is so your doctor can observe and assess the progression of your healing and recovery, answer any questions you may have and make adjustments to medications or physical therapy.

Ask your advocate to go with you to the first post-surgical follow-up visit with your surgeon so they can also hear the next set of recommendations for your recovery. It's a good idea to have an extra set of ears with you for this step. An advocate can help you remember to ask questions you may have and can write down follow-up care instructions while you speak with the doctor.

If you have pressing questions that you'd like answered before your scheduled follow-up visit, call your surgeon's office and get them answered. This is something your doctor and his office staff are there to assist you with.

PART II:

IF YOU HAVE TIME TO PLAN AND PREPARE

1: HOW DO YOU PREPARE FOR SURGERY?

How do you eat an elephant?
One bite at a time.
How do you prepare for surgery?
One step at a time!

■ ■ ■

While Part I of this book applies to everyone having planned or unplanned surgery, Part II is designed for those who have advance notice of surgery, to help navigate often complicated and confusing territory. If you're in the decision-making process prior to committing to surgery, there can be a lot of information to collect and wrap your brain around. Preparing and taking the steps to get ready is valuable, but can feel overwhelming, especially if you are scared, don't feel well or are in pain. Take a moment and simply acknowledge that.

With that in mind, given time and the opportunity,

Any time and effort spent preparing yourself before surgery
will positively influence your experience and recovery.

The checklists on the following pages will help guide you through the planning, preparation and surgery experience. Have a pen ready to take notes on additional insights and ideas that spring to mind as you read. A great tool to begin with is a dedicated notebook.

Dedicate a spiral notebook, 3-ring binder or even a phone app to keep track of notes, questions and all things surgery related. With everything written down in one place, it's easy to locate information, review notes or refresh your memory if you forget something. Pick a system that is easy for you and then stick with it; consistency is helpful. If you can, set this system up before surgery. If not, ask someone to help you organize notes and create a system once you're home from the hospital.

A NOTEBOOK/MEDICAL JOURNAL IS A GREAT PLACE TO:

- **Keep track of all procedure-related information**. Doctor, nurse and scheduler names and contact information and doctor visit notes. Writing down what you hear at appointments will allow you to remember what has been said, by whom and when.[xxiii] This is really helpful when a lot of information is given all at once.
- **Take notes on impressions of individuals, faculties and treatment options**.
- **Write down questions that come to mind or things you want to remember**.
- **Create checklists to ensure things get accomplished before surgery**.
- **Track your progress**. With a progress log, you can look back and see when, where and how you are improving and all the milestones you've hit along the way. Being able to refer back to a progress log is especially helpful when you feel stuck or like you aren't progressing or getting better.
- **Write post-surgery notes.** Designate an area in your notebook for post-surgery notes. Following surgery, you may be fuzzy so notes can be helpful and provide a snapshot of: (1) medications you've taken and when, (2) what you've eaten and when, (3) when you were last out of bed and moving around, (4) when you last used the bathroom and (5) when you last applied ice, for example.

[xxiii] You can also audio-record conversations for exact details, if that would be easier or helpful for you.

ORGANIZING YOUR MEDICAL FILES

. . .

With your written notes all in one place, next consider creating a dedicated medical file (or system) for other pertinent procedure-related information. (I personally think accordion files are great for keeping things categorized and organized.[xxiv]) With everything located in one place, it's easy to find and access information and it's also easy to grab information if needed when heading out the door to a doctor appointment.

ITEMS TO INCLUDE IN YOUR MEDICAL FILE:

☐ **A copy of your insurance card(s)**, front and back.

☐ **Doctor, surgeon, hospital (or surgical center) names and contact information**. (See template on pages 178.)

☐ **Your emergency contact information.** Family members, friends, neighbors, advocate, etc. (See template on pages 178-179.)

☐ **A copy of your personal information (blood type, allergies, intolerances, sensitivities), medical history and hospitalizations.** Include all previous surgeries, injuries, illnesses and hospitalizations. (See templates on pages 176 and 177.)

☐ **A list of current medications, vitamins, minerals, herbs you are taking and your dosing schedule.** (See templates on pages 180 and 181.)

☐ **X-ray, MRI, ultrasound, electrocardiogram (EKG) films and reports.** These days, copies of X-rays, MRIs and radiology reports can easily be loaded onto a CD that you can take with you. (No more bulky X-ray negatives that need to be signed out and returned.) Whenever you have an X-ray taken, be sure to ask for copies of the images and reports for your files.

☐ **Copies of blood work or other lab and test results.**

☐ **Other procedure-related documents or information.** For example, copies of any research you may have collected.

☐ **Pre- and post-surgery instructions and follow-up directions**; these should be provided by your surgeon.

[xxiv] Note: Pages 176-186 contain templates to help organize information including: medical history and hospitalizations, medications being taken, emergency contact information, doctor appointment notes, daily progress notes, pain management tracking, people who have offered to help and more. A sample Living Will can be found on pages 192-193. Free .DOCX and .PDF downloads of each template are also available at LORIMERTZ.COM/FREE-DOWNLOADS.HTML.

☐ **Physical therapy notes and home exercises.**

☐ **Medical receipts, bills and invoices.** This is important so you can review bills for accuracy (make sure there are no overcharges) and track expenses that: (1) will be reimbursed by your insurance company or (2) are out of your pocket (such as co-pays or any uncovered devices, wound care, dressing products, etc.). You may also want to keep a budget in this file. Basic home budgeting principles are important during this time so that stress about finances doesn't get added to the list of things on your mind.

CHOOSING YOUR EXPERIENCE

Choosing your experience is about honoring yourself and being empowered in your choices.
You are choosing to have surgery.
You are choosing the surgeon you want.

∎ ∎ ∎

Where do you start? You start with the first step. We all know what we don't want. The trick is to get clear on what we DO want and focus on it, so we can have that experience.

GET CLEAR AND SET YOUR INTENTIONS

- What does your ideal surgical experience look like to you?
- How does it feel to you?
- Who's with you?
- Do you feel safe with your doctor, surgeon and medical team? If you get a 'no' feeling, you can make a change at any time, for any reason. *This is your surgery and your decision*; it doesn't have to make sense to anyone but you *it's about you and how you feel.*
- Is your procedure being performed in a hospital or surgical center? Do you feel comfortable and relaxed there? For example, when I had back surgery it was an out-patient procedure and I was given several hospital and surgical center options. After checking them out, I chose the place I felt the most comfortable and at ease.

ALLOW FOR YOUR UNIQUE RIGHT TIMING—CHOOSE TO TAKE YOUR TIME

As patients, we understandably want to know definitive timetables for healing and recovery and it can feel frustrating when doctors or physical therapists are wobbly on this. The amount of time it takes to return to "normal" is going to be different for everybody and every body. Recovery time can be faster for some patients (especially those in good physical shape with youth on their side) and slower for others (such as people who are older or who smoke, drink alcohol, are overweight or out of shape), but there is no way to tell definitively. Choose to allow your healing—your timing—to unfold rather than trying to force it based on a "should" or someone else's timing.

This is the right time to take your time and take it easy.
You are worth it!

Be prepared to spend time resting and mending. Listen to and follow doctors' directions. In addition, check in and listen to yourself and your body. Notice changes, big or small. Pay attention to and acknowledge even small decreases in pain as well as increases in energy and activity; these are signs that healing and recovery are taking place.

Pushing yourself too hard or too fast before or after surgery may cause setbacks in the healing and recovery process. Again, healing simply takes as long as it takes. There is no magic bullet, pill or formula, it's just one step—one day—at a time.

"It's a matter of timing and patience.
Although it may seem nothing is happening on the surface,
there may be profound changes occurring a little deeper. Waiting isn't bad."
Buck Brannaman

TRUST YOUR INSTINCTS

Your instincts are there to keep you safe and are sending signals (feelings, intuitions, spontaneous insights) to protect you. Notice thoughts or feelings you have. Pay attention, listen and take action. Trust yourself.

SEE IT THROUGH

> *Your recovery,*
> *your health and*
> *your well-being*
> *are the foundation*
> *of your entire life.*

Since you're committing to and undertaking the time and expense to have surgery, honor those commitments and see it through. Why jeopardize your long-term outcome with short-term impatience? What's one more day of rest or one more day away from work when examined in the context of an entire lifetime?

HEALING TAKES AS LONG AS IT TAKES, QUICKER FOR SOME, SLOWER FOR OTHERS

When a woman I know fell and broke seven ribs and punctured a lung, even after time in the hospital, a month at a rehab facility and months resting and taking it easy, over a year later she continued to notice improvements in her energy level and ability to move around and lift things. Healing was a much longer, and sometimes much more frustrating, process than she anticipated, realized or was prepared for; she just wanted to get back to her regular routine.

Again, healing simply takes as long as it takes; quicker for some, slower for others. Try not to judge your healing pace, just allow it to unfold.

GET ENROLLED—ASK WHY—QUESTION EVERYTHING

*It is our job to make sure we get all the information we need
to make solid and informed decisions about our health.*

■ ■ ■

As a surgical patient, you are "going under the knife," literally and figuratively, in some way. I believe an important component in preparing for surgery (or any major life event) is our own enrollment in the process. With regard to surgery, doctors can be great at telling us what to do for our health, but may fail to explain or communicate *why* what they say or recommend is important.

For me, knowing the "why" behind the "what" enrolls me in doing what has been recommended. Following directions is easy, but if I know "why" I'm doing something and "how" it's valuable to and impacting me, then I'm more motivated and invested and likelier to follow through. Don't give your power away by just doing what someone—a doctor, for example—says. Knowing why can make a difference. **Ask questions. Learn why.**

TIPS:

☐ Be inquisitive. Ask why a recommendation is being made.

☐ Ask questions until you understand and feel satisfied, comfortable and confident with the answers before moving forward. There have been many times when I've asked a doctor a question and not understood their answer and had to ask them—several times even—for clarification. "I'm sorry, I heard what you said, but I didn't get it. Can you please explain it in a different way?" **A good doctor will patiently explain something until you understand.**

■ ■ ■

A FEW EXAMPLES WHERE KNOWING "WHY" MAY MAKE A DIFFERENCE

Don't eat or drink the night before surgery. Okay, but why is that really important?
Anesthesia can cause nausea and vomiting which can aspirate any food or liquid in your stomach to the lungs, possibly causing serious complications or even death in extreme cases. To be safe, don't eat or drink anything 10-12 hours prior to surgery, or as directed by your anesthesiologist.

What about just sucking on a mint or chewing gum?

Good question. Nope, not even these. The action of sucking on candy or chewing gum sends a message to the stomach to prepare for food, which causes the stomach to generate digestive liquids, which should be avoided for the same reason as above.

Tell your doctor everything (prescription medications, over-the-counter drugs, vitamins, minerals, herbs, recreational drugs) you're taking before surgery. Why?

It may be important to discontinue some substances prior to surgery. Things like over-the-counter aspirin, ibuprofen and naproxen, Alka-Seltzer products, Pepto-Bismol, the herb ginseng, vitamin E and others may cause bleeding problems or other complications during or after surgery. To avoid negative interactions or complications, it's best to disclose everything you are taking and follow your doctor's directions on their use (or discontinuation of) prior to and after surgery.

Be sure and get extra sleep. Okay, why?

Among other benefits, the restorative growth hormone required for healing is primarily released when you reach deep stage three/stage four sleep. This is just one reason it's important to sleep—and sleep well—prior to and following surgery. (See pages 72-76 for more about sleeping and resting and their importance.)

Stop smoking. Okay, but why?

In short, because smoking can cause complications, delay healing and interfere with the actions of certain drugs. The most common complications related to smoking are: (1) delayed or impaired wound and tissue healing, (2) greater scarring, (3) wound infection, (4) cardiopulmonary complications (smokers are at greater risk for requiring the ventilator for longer periods of time) and (5) possible interference with the actions of certain drugs. Not smoking (even cutting back) will allow lungs to work better which will improve blood flow and circulation, sweeping debris away from the incision site, helping you to heal.

Meet With Your Surgeon

. . .

If possible, arrange to see your surgeon several weeks before your scheduled procedure. In addition to getting your questions answered, this is when your surgeon will determine and advise you of any labs, x-rays, appointments or clearances that may be required before your surgery. Schedule these items well in advance so there is plenty of time to get the results in hand and have them reviewed. Having things taken care of early in the process can prevent stressful last-minute rushing around. Learning about your surgery in advance will also allow you to get mentally, emotionally and physically prepared for the surgery, recovery and any follow up treatments, hopefully alleviating some worrying caused by the unknown.

MAKE TIME WITH YOUR DOCTOR COUNT

Bring a written list of questions to your appointment. Since time with your surgeon may be limited, prioritizing questions can be helpful, too. Some offices may prefer you email or fax your questions ahead of time; ask. Bring your notebook, pen and advocate (or second set of ears[xxv]) to this meeting as well. Listen, take notes and get the information you need to feel safe and confident. (See sample questions for your surgeon on pages 128-129 and a list of things you may want to share or discuss with your surgeon on pages 130-135.)

TRUST, BUT VERIFY—GET A SECOND OPINION

Getting a second opinion is for your safety and is valuable because different surgeons may have different approaches to the same surgery. They will also have different personalities; one surgeon may put you more at ease than another. Hearing from more than one professional will provide a helpful comparison on surgical approaches and personalities.

For example, a highly regarded surgeon, who I really liked and felt comfortable with, said I was going to need back surgery. To explore what other options might exist, I got a second opinion. The surgeon I went to for the second opinion happened to also be nice and patiently answered all my questions. As it turned out, he recommended the exact same procedure. Knowing that I was going to use the first

---

[xxv] Refer to pages 5-9 for valuable information about advocates, an essential resource to have throughout all stages of the surgical process, before surgery, at the hospital and after surgery.

neurosurgeon I'd met, I confessed to the second doctor that I had come to him for a second opinion. He acknowledged that getting a second opinion was a smart idea.

If for some reason you still have lingering questions or doubts, even after meeting with two surgeons, honor yourself and get a third opinion. I have a friend who tore his Achilles tendon playing basketball and he actually interviewed four different surgeons before making his final choice.

QUESTIONS TO ASK YOUR SURGEON

Get clear about the benefits, risks and possible complications of the proposed surgery. Take notes on impressions and details. Whether you're interviewing prospective surgeons or meeting with the surgeon you've chosen, the following are some questions you may want to ask. (Note: Many doctors are affiliated with clinics that have websites that may be able to answer some of your questions.)

QUESTIONS ABOUT THE SURGEON'S CREDENTIALS:

- ☐ Are you board certified in a surgical specialty? How many years?
- ☐ How many patients have you treated with my particular problem?
- ☐ How often do you perform *this* procedure?
- ☐ What is your experience and track record with this procedure?

QUESTIONS ABOUT THE SURGERY/PROCEDURE:

- ☐ What operation are you recommending? What is the exact name of the procedure?
- ☐ Why do I need this operation?
- ☐ What are the benefits? In what ways will my life be different after this procedure?
- ☐ What are the risks, possible complications or downsides? Can I lessen these?
- ☐ Is this the procedure you'd recommend if I were your spouse/child/parent?
- ☐ Is this surgery absolutely necessary? Are there any alternatives to surgery?
- ☐ Is there more than one surgical approach to what I need?
- ☐ Is this procedure a "cure" or a temporary "fix"? How long will the benefits last?
- ☐ What if I choose not to have this operation? What are the ramifications?
- ☐ Is it important or time-sensitive to have this surgery done right now or can I elect to have it at another time?
- ☐ Where will the operation be performed? Do I get a choice of locations?
- ☐ Will this be an out-patient or in-patient procedure? How long will I be in the hospital?
- ☐ How will my other (unrelated) health care needs be managed during and after surgery? (For example, if a patient requires special medication, insulin, etc.)
- ☐ What kind of scarring can I expect?
- ☐ Could I need a transfusion? (See page 136 for information on blood donation.)
- ☐ Can I get a prescription for pre-hab? (See pages 143-144 for more on pre-hab.)

- ☐ Will you be performing the procedure at a teaching hospital? If yes, ask who will be doing your actual procedure. Note: If you are uncomfortable with anyone other than your surgeon working on you, it is important to verbalize this. For example, when I had open-heart surgery, it was performed at Massachusetts General Hospital in Boston, which is a teaching hospital for Harvard medical students. Before surgery, my mother (and advocate) was extremely clear with my surgeon, he was the only doctor authorized to perform the surgery. He confirmed "yes," it would be only him, not a student or fellow. He did request permission to have students observe, which I agreed to.

QUESTIONS ABOUT ANESTHESIA:

- ☐ What type of anesthesia will I be given?
- ☐ What are the risks and side effects?
- ☐ Do I have a choice of which type of anesthesia I will be given: general, regional or local? (See page 159 for an explanation of each method.)
- ☐ Note: If you've had previous negative experiences with anesthesia, you may be required to make an appointment for evaluation by an anesthesiologist prior surgery.

POST-SURGERY QUESTIONS:

- ☐ How long is the recovery for this particular procedure? What should I expect?
- ☐ What does a "normal" recovery look like?
- ☐ Are there any special instructions that can help speed my recovery?
- ☐ Will I need things like oxygen or assistive devices (crutches, braces, slings, etc.)?
- ☐ What prescriptions will I need to take after surgery? Why? For how long?
- ☐ Can I fill prescriptions prior to surgery so they are available when I get home?
- ☐ Will I need in-patient rehabilitation? If yes, do I get to choose the facility? How can I get more information about this?
- ☐ Will I need home health services during my recovery? Who arranges this? Is it covered by my insurance?
- ☐ What physical limitations will I have after surgery? For how long?
- ☐ Will I need physical therapy following surgery? For approximately how long?
- ☐ When can I get back to my "normal" activities such as work, exercise, sex, other?

ADDITIONAL QUESTIONS:

- ☐ _____
- ☐ _____
- ☐ _____

THINGS TO SHARE AND DISCUSS WITH
YOUR SURGEON BEFORE SURGERY

Once you've decided to have surgery and have chosen a surgeon, there are many things you may want to discuss with your surgeon before surgery. Being thorough is for your safety and peace of mind.

ALLERGIES

Disclose and remind doctors, nurses and health care providers of any allergies you have. Include food, drug and environmental allergies; allergies to things such as latex, tape or Neosporin. Include allergies to things you don't think could possibly matter. For example, an egg allergy, which may not seem pertinent when having surgery, is indeed important because many medications are formulated in an egg base, which can be significant in a highly sensitive patient. Nothing is inconsequential.[xxvi]

If your allergy is life-threatening, remain vigilant. In spite of best efforts (communicating, having notes written in your chart and wearing a special allergy alert bracelet), allergies far too often get missed. I have many firsthand experiences with family members and friends who have had close calls.

My mom, for example, has a significant allergy to penicillin and any penicillin derivative. In spite of her diligence and constant reminders to doctors, on one occasion, even though she'd carefully explained how deathly allergic she is to penicillin and its derivatives, a doctor wrote her a prescription for a medication containing penicillin. While the doctor assured her she had nothing to worry about, because of her previous experiences, prior to filling the prescription she called her pharmacist to double-check the ingredients. The pharmacist confirmed her suspicion, "yes," the prescription *did* contain a 10% penicillin derivative, which is enough to possibly kill her.

This is why advocates and advocating for ourselves is so crucial. No one is infallible, including our doctor.

[xxvi] Note: Most people usually find out they have allergies because they have had an allergic reaction such as an itchy rash, blisters or hives, hay fever, runny nose or nasal congestion, watery itchy eyes, scratchy throat, sneezing, coughing, wheezing, difficulty breathing or worse. Among other things, doctors and nurses are keen observers and hopefully notice if a patient has an unexpected allergic reaction to something.

Medications, vitamins, minerals and herbs taken regularly

For your safety, your doctor and surgeon need to know the name, strength, dosage and frequency of any medication (prescription or over-the-counter) or supplement you take. The reason for a detailed disclosure is that some medications and products can cause interactions or complications during surgery. Be sure to include products that you might not think are important such as aspirin, ibuprofen, diet pills, vitamins, minerals, herbs, even protein powders. Ask which you should discontinue the days or weeks prior to surgery and verify what you can begin retaking following surgery, and when. Being thorough is for your safety. Some complications can be serious, but may be avoidable.

Creating this list *prior* to doctor appointments will eliminate having to remember this information when asked at appointments. (Use the templates on pages 180 and 181 to help you organize this information.)

Recreational drug use

Recreational drugs include "legal" and "illegal" drugs such as alcohol, cigarettes or marijuana, prescription or over-the-counter drugs, cocaine, heroin, meth, crack, etc. These products can cause negative drug interactions or complications. (See pages 146-148 for more on substances that can negatively affect surgery and recovery.)

Religious preferences

This may be important, as it can affect treatment options. Alerting doctors to the fact that you cannot receive blood for religious reasons, for example, is vital information to communicate. With this information, doctors and surgeons can create an alternative plan that takes into account and respects religious beliefs.

Dental work

Mention dental work or dental care (of any kind) that you may be having prior to or just following your surgery. ***Some dental procedures can increase the risk of complications and should be rescheduled.*** Even a simple routine cleaning can cause bacteria to be dislodged and enter the blood stream, possibly causing infection.

Get a written list of do's and don'ts following surgery

Advance notice of any post-surgical restrictions can help you prepare for and organize your post-surgery life and schedule.

Ask if you may require extended in-patient rehab

Sometimes a transitional stay in a rehabilitation facility is necessary if patients are too weak to care for themselves or their home cannot accommodate their needs. This is especially true for older or less mobile patients. The hospital may have such a unit or have a relationship with a nearby rehabilitation facility. If you are in the hospital when this need arises, the hospital social worker will meet with you and discuss available options before any decision or transfer is made; you will make any final decision.

If you know in advance that you may require extended in-patient rehab, you may wish to do some research. Services and specialties vary among rehab centers along with a facilities "look" and "feel." Different centers may also take different insurance and have different co-pays. Get recommendations from your doctor, physical therapists or friends who have had recent stays and come up with a plan you are comfortable with in the event you require an extended stay prior to going home.

Illness

Notify your surgeon if you develop a fever, cold, rash or other new symptom prior to surgery, even if it seems insignificant to you. For your safety, it may be necessary to postpone and reschedule the procedure.

Driving

After surgery there are usually guidelines as to when a patient can safely get back behind the wheel of a car. It may be as soon as a day or two or significantly longer, as in the case of abdominal or thoracic surgery or surgery involving the right leg or hip. *Driving too soon following surgery can jeopardize both you and others.*

For example, following surgery, a patients' response time may be delayed due to pain or pain medications, causing an unwanted accident. A jarring move in a car could also jeopardize a tender surgical repair that needs protecting. Drivers beware: some automobile insurance policies include clauses that restrict post-surgical driving, invalidating a policy in the event of an accident.

For me, following reconstructive surgery on my left knee, even though I was cleared to drive, I was strictly forbidden to place any pressure on my left leg for several months, which left me unable to drive my standard transmission (stick shift) car. Unfortunately this didn't occur to me prior to surgery and no one mentioned it. Knowing this ahead of time would have been very helpful so I could have planned ahead. Luckily, a friend generously traded me her automatic for several months until I could safely drive my own car again. Thank you, Beck!

Do you need a temporary handicap parking placard or permit? If yes, there is a form that your surgeon will fill out which will then need to be taken to your local Department of Motor Vehicles (DMV) who will issue the placard for you. Note: Procedures for getting a temporary handicap placard vary from state to state. For example, in some states AAA (American Automobile Association) can take the completed form and issue the parking placard. Ask your doctor, call the DMV or search the Internet to find out for sure.

POST-SURGICAL ASSISTIVE DEVICES

Assistive devices required following surgery (such as crutches following knee surgery or a walker following a hip replacement) should be provided for you at the hospital or surgical center prior to discharge. In some cases assistive devices such as a continuous passive motion machine (see image on page 135) may be delivered and set up by a home health agency once you are home. If you will need non-medically necessary devices, such as an electric reclining chair, bedside commode or shower chair following surgery, try and get them before surgery, if possible. Having them on hand and ready when you get home from the hospital or surgical center will be helpful.

Ask your doctor or their staff for recommendations on where to rent or purchase medical equipment, or, get creative. For example, a stable plastic chair on a rubber shower mat may be a suitable less expensive substitute for a shower chair (see image on page 30). I have found AMAZON.COM to be a good resource for most anything these days.

If the patient is over 50 years old, local senior centers[xxvii] can be valuable resources for assistive device rentals such as wheelchairs, walkers, canes, shower chairs and commodes. For example, the Oasis Senior Center in Corona del Mar, California rents all of the above for $1.00 a month.

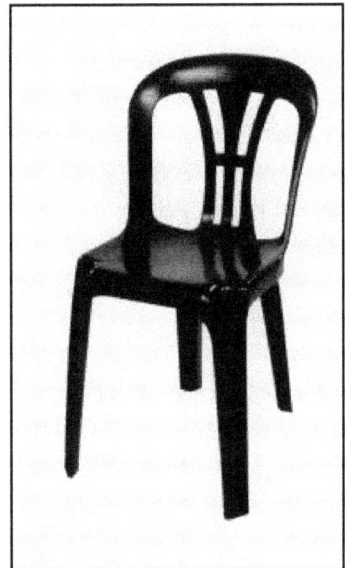

[xxvii] Senior centers may additionally have excellent gyms, classes and libraries. They can be wonderful and valuable resources.

Be aware, some insurance companies do not cover some assistive devices (such as shower chairs or other non-medically necessary equipment), so verify coverage with your insurance company and then, if necessary, plan for this expense. If your insurance covers post-surgical assistive devices, be aware that you may need a prescription from your doctor to receive reimbursement.

ASSISTIVE DEVICE EXAMPLES:

- **Wheelchair**. Will you temporarily need a transport (lightweight and made for others to push you) or manual (self-propelling) wheelchair?
- **Walker**. Consider getting a basket for the front to carry items when you move from one room to another.
- **Crutches**
- **Cane** (there are many styles: standard, straight-handled, broad-based)
- **Bedside commode**
- **Raised toilet seat** (See image on page 30.)
- **Shower chair** (See image on page 30.)
- **Reclining chair with electric lift**. These chairs can be especially helpful after back, spine, neck or abdominal surgery. A reclining chair can be adjusted to optimize comfort and reduce pain, allowing for quality rest or sleep. An electric lift can also assist in standing, actually lifting you to your feet. I have a friend who used one after a hysterectomy and she said that it was the only place she could get comfortable and sleep. (It was a month before she was able sleep in her own bed again.)

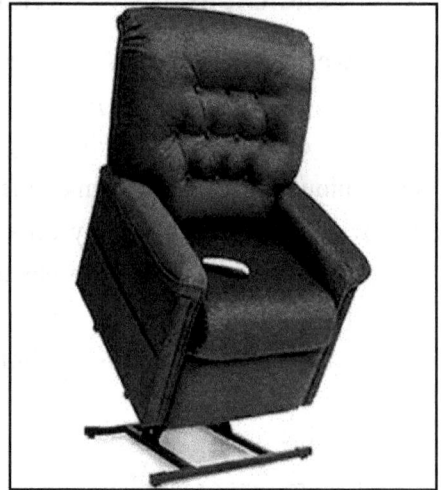
Electric Reclining Chair

- **Cold therapy unit**. Often used after orthopedic surgery, it's a cooler-like device with a motorized pump providing continuous cold-water circulation to an extremity via tubing and a bladder. I found this device to be comfortable and easy to use when I was in bed. When I found myself in another room, rather than moving the unit, a bag of frozen peas was an easy alternative.

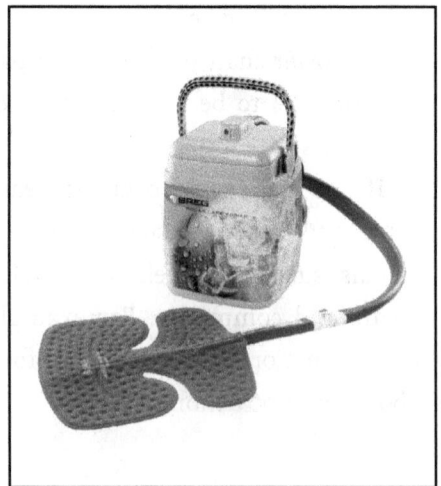
Cold Therapy Unit

- **Continuous passive motion machine**. These are used to gently flex and extend joints after some orthopedic procedures. I had one after knee surgery and think it aided my recovery. Some doctors use them, some don't. It seems to be a matter of opinion.

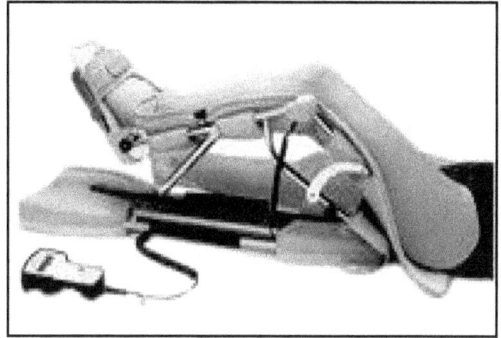

Continuous Passive Motion Machine

ADDITIONAL QUESTIONS:

- ☐ _____
  _____
- ☐ _____
  _____
- ☐ _____
  _____
- ☐ _____
  _____

THINGS THAT REQUIRE PLANNING BEFORE SURGERY

Depending on the procedure you are undergoing, there may be some standard medical clearances, tests or x-rays that your doctor will need you to complete prior to surgery. If anything is required, your doctor will provide a prescription and referral.

- ☐ **Physical exam and health clearances**. Some surgeons may require some surgical patients to have a physical exam or obtain other health clearances prior to surgery.
- ☐ **Blood tests and lab work**
- ☐ **X-rays, MRI, CAT scan, ultrasound, electrocardiogram (EKG), etc**. Note: If you need and MRI and are at all claustrophobic, be sure to mention this to your doctor and at upon check-in when you get your MRI.
- ☐ **Do you need to meet with the anesthesiologist to discuss anesthesia methods or prior difficulties with anesthesia?** (See anesthesia methods on pages 159-160.)
- ☐ **Blood donation**. Is it possible you may need a blood transfusion? If the answer is 'yes,' ask about donating your own blood (autologous blood donation) prior to surgery Why? Although the blood supply available today is considered very safe, receiving your own blood is the safest and most compatible blood for you.

  The benefits to receiving your own blood include: (1) no risk of reaction to foreign antigens—your body recognizes its own blood and readily accepts it and (2) no possibility of disease being transmitted from the blood of another person.

  If you prefer to receive your own blood, be sure you speak up for it. Because it is more work, oftentimes doctors and hospitals will attempt to persuade you to receive blood bank blood. Be clear and stick to your guns about things that you believe in and feel strongly about.

  To begin the process of autologous donation, your physician's office must send an order to the hospital or surgical center where your surgery is taking place. You can then go to that facility and donate. Autologous blood donations require planning and need to be made 3-5 days in advance of surgery. (Note: People who aren't able to donate blood for others may still be able to donate blood for themselves.)

Questions To Ask Hospital or Surgical Center
Staff, Schedulers and Social Workers

Schedulers, social workers and other key hospital staff members may be of assistance in getting general questions answered or determining what benefits you may be eligible for such as insurance, government benefits or other programs.

Questions about financial stuff

☐ Do I qualify for Medicare or Medicaid?

☐ Does being a war veteran entitle me to any special health care benefits?

☐ Do I qualify for any financial assistance or other hospital programs?

☐ If I am self-paying, can I pay the insurance rate? Is there a special discount plan or installment program available for self-paying patients?

☐ Is this hospital and *all* its providers, services, equipment, etc. covered by my health insurance? What exactly will I be expected to pay out-of-pocket?

☐ If needed after my procedure, who will be assisting me in finding and making arrangements with a rehabilitation facility or home health care agency? Will I get a choice of where I go? Will the cost be the same or different at various facilities?

General

☐ I would like to tour the hospital (or surgical center). When can we set this up?

☐ Is it okay if someone (advocate, friend or family member) stays overnight in the hospital with me? *If this is important to you, ask what needs to be done in order to accommodate this request!*

☐ Do you have generic advance directive templates such as Special Power of Attorney or Living Will I can use? (See pages 188-191 for more on these topics and a sample Living Will).

Additional questions:

☐ _____
_____

☐ _____
_____

☐ _____
_____

GET CLEAR ABOUT INSURANCE COVERAGE

■ ■ ■

Given time to plan and prepare for surgery, or any procedure, it is crucial to talk with your insurance company. Get clear on your coverage and any expenses you may be personally responsible for paying. To ensure coverage, a non-emergency procedure *must be pre-authorized* by your insurance company. Most surgeries (with the exception of most cosmetic surgeries) are covered in some part by health insurance (if you have it). In most cases your doctor or surgeon will get the necessary insurance pre-authorizations for you, but independently verify this information for your peace of mind. For example, sometimes a patient will receive separate bills from their surgeon, surgical assistant, anesthesiologist, hospital or surgical center and any other specialty physicians or medical equipment suppliers. In this case, each of these providers would need to be pre-approved.

QUESTION EVERYTHING

Asking a lot of questions upfront can help prevent financial surprises down the road. There may be nuances in your insurance policy that are important to understand before scheduling a procedure. For example, unless there are extenuating circumstances, some surgeries or procedures may only be covered as an out-patient procedure. In such a case, you might choose to have that procedure done at an out-patient surgical center rather than hospital to avoid being responsible for additional charges.

DOCUMENT EVERYTHING

Document conversations with your insurance company in the event questions arise later. Write down the date, name and extension of each representative you speak with and the outcome of each conversation. Write down what your coverage provides and allows for and what your financial responsibility or co-pay will be. Verify that the surgical facility (hospital or surgical center) and each of the individuals (surgeon, anesthesiologist, etc.) and medical equipment suppliers involved in your care will be covered by your insurance and whether they are covered as in-network, or out-of-network providers. Understand your deductible and your co-pays; 80/20, 70/30, 60/40 or 50/50.

To avoid any confusion regarding coverage after the fact, *get authorization from your insurance company in writing*. Having this information upfront, and in writing, can eliminate stressful financial surprises down the road, which are not helpful during the healing process.

CASES IN POINT

I have heard stories about doctor's offices telling patients they are covered, but it later turns out the authorization was only for the doctor, not the anesthesiologist, surgical center or other departments. I've also heard stories about insurance companies approving preventive care procedures, then, after the procedure, saying that a patient had already met their preventive care allotment for the year, so the procedure was, in fact, not covered. I have a friend who was told his co-pay would be $149 for a preventive colonoscopy, only to find out later that was only for the doctor's fee; it didn't include the anesthesiologist's fee or surgical center fee. Each case ultimately got resolved, but each one took a great deal of time and energy. Mistakes happen, but it's easier to avoid these pitfalls with some extra due diligence on the front end, if possible.

Again, being clear and well educated on what your policy covers can help prevent surprise bills and frustrating experiences down the road.

WHAT IF I DON'T HAVE INSURANCE COVERAGE?

If you are an uninsured patient, one thing to remember is: *Everything is negotiable.*

If possible (if you are having planned vs. unplanned surgery), get thorough estimates upfront. It's sort of like bidding for a job or contract at work or purchasing a new car. Generate a list of what you want and need and then get several estimates. Be sure that when you get quotes you are comparing apples to apples, that each estimate includes all the same services.

Some hospitals have become very transparent in this respect and have begun posting their rates online. For example, The Surgery Center of Oklahoma (SURGERYCENTEROK.COM) offers detailed upfront pricing for cash patients for many different surgical procedures, both in- and out-patient.

Prescription medications are another item that can vary drastically in price from one pharmacy to another. I have seen the price of a prescription medication differ as much as $100, sometimes more. I have also noticed a significant difference in prices from state-to-state. This seems to be especially true for brand name pharmaceuticals vs. generic brands.

Again, as you create your estimate, be sure you know exactly what you need and carefully observe what is—and what is not—included in the pricing doctors and institutions give you.

Questions To Ask Your Insurance Company

- ☐ Am I covered for this procedure?
- ☐ Is my surgeon covered?
- ☐ Is the anesthesiologist covered?
- ☐ Is the hospital or surgical center covered?
- ☐ How much will it cost me after insurance pays its portion?
- ☐ What is the maximum out-of-pocket I should expect to pay for this procedure?
- ☐ What is the maximum coverage allowed by my policy? Will this procedure hit that?
- ☐ Is in-patient rehabilitation or home health care covered after surgery if needed?
- ☐ Is my physical therapy covered? How many visits am I allowed under my policy? What if I require additional physical therapy?
- ☐ If I need special equipment after surgery, such as oxygen, braces, crutches, continuous passive motion machine, wheelchair, hospital bed, bedside commode, walker, cane, shower chair or other assistive device, are they covered?
- ☐ What is my prescription coverage?
- ☐ Is there anything else I should know or be aware of?
- ☐ **Please send me this approval in writing.**

ADDITIONAL QUESTIONS:

- ☐ _____
  _____
- ☐ _____
  _____
- ☐ _____
  _____
- ☐ _____
  _____

Again, to avoid anxiety or financial surprises, verify the level of health care coverage you have prior to undergoing any procedure, surgery or treatment (if possible) so you are fully aware of any medical bills or co-pays that you will be responsible for and expected to pay out-of-pocket.

Prepare For Work Absence

*Your health is the foundation
upon which everything else in your life is built.*

■ ■ ■

If you work, and have time to plan ahead prior to surgery, there are things you may be able to do to prepare yourself for work absence. Being organized for the time away from work can allow for peace of mind, which will, in turn, allow you to channel your energy into the more important job at hand—your health and your recovery. While some are anxious to get back to work quickly, if you return to work too soon, it may compromise both your on-going recovery and your work performance.

Ideas for preparing for work absence

In general, ask questions. Ascertain eligibility and follow through with paperwork.

- ☐ **Schedule time to be gone with your boss and human resources**. The human resources department is designed to help you get answers to questions concerning your job and benefits.
- ☐ **Verify and clarify absence benefits**. Ask about the use of unused sick leave, vacation time, personal time and short- and long-term benefits. Ask if your job will be held if there are complications and you require additional unforeseen recovery time.
- ☐ **Familiarize yourself with the Family Medical Leave Act (FMLA)**. If you are anxious about getting back to work to ensure your position, check into your rights; the FMLA is there in the event of a medical emergency (your own, or that of a family member).

  The FMLA is a federal law that lets qualified employees take extended time away from work in the event of an emergency. It provides employees unpaid, job-protected leave (all at once or intermittently) if you are unable to work because of your own serious health condition, or because you need to care for a parent, spouse or child. Visit the United States Department of Labor website, DOL.GOV/WHD/FMLA, for details, requirements, qualifications and additional information, and speak with your employer. In addition, many states have laws that may provide coverage above and beyond that outlined in the FMLA.
- ☐ **Ask about insurance payments that need to be made in your absence** so your policy stays current.

☐ **Prepare for time away.** If you know you are going to be out of the office, cover yourself. If possible, create a plan with your co-workers so you don't return to a heap of emails, voicemails or projects needing your immediate attention. With a little planning, it is possible to unplug.

☐ **Don't go back to work too soon.** Following any procedure, your body is going to be stressed and tired. You've been through the hardest part, why risk your recovery now? Instead, allow yourself and your body time to really rest and heal properly and completely. While it may not seem like it, life can and will carry on without you for a stint.

If you must, bring a little work home to keep you occupied. If you don't already have a laptop computer, ask your company if you can borrow one. But really, forget work. The more important job at hand is you. Healing simply takes time. Patience and time.

☐ **When it's time, ease back into work.** When you think you are physically ready to go back to work, consider easing into your regular work routine. See if it's possible to begin by working part-time from home, or with short days in the office. Gradually increase your schedule as you feel stronger.

To conserve energy, arrange for a spouse, friend or co-worker to drive you to and from work. Even when you're feeling better, healing is still taking place.

It is worth noting that a full recovery—one where you feel back to your pre-surgery self—can take months. Healing continues long after a scab has dried up and fallen off or a cast is removed. If your injury is severe, or the surgery is really involved, it could take up to a year or longer. For me, healing from my head injury was years. For my friend who fell, much to her dismay, healing from seven broken ribs and a punctured lung took over a year. My friend who had major lung surgery is currently in her twelfth post-operative month and while she is back at work and doing well, there are still days she simply needs to stay home and rest.

☐ **On the other hand, if you're unhappy at your current job, you may wish to use your time in bed to work on your resumé.** Surf the net, call headhunters, explore other options.

ADDITIONAL QUESTIONS:

☐ _____

_____

☐ _____

_____

GET PRE-HAB

■ ■ ■

It's a new word, but a groovy and valuable concept. Pre-hab—pre-habilitation—is an exercise therapy and strengthening program started weeks, or even months, before surgery if possible, safe and recommended by your doctor. Rather than just depending on your surgeon to fix you up, given the luxury of advance notice before surgery, any physical preparation—pre-hab—will positively affect your post-surgical outcome and recovery.

Why is it valuable? The stronger you go into surgery, the stronger you'll come out and the faster you will be able to get back to your day-to-day activities. Patients who are active and fit before surgery may have shorter hospital stays and are often able to go home for out-patient rehab, rather than be discharged to an in-patient rehab facility.

I have experienced the value of pre-hab first-hand and it works. Statistics and doctors reinforce that experience.

> *"Fifty percent of (surgical) outcome success is due to the surgeon, and the other 50% is due to the patient's commitment to recovery—starting with pre-hab. Pre-hab makes a huge difference in our patients' outcomes. They get vertical sooner and recover faster."*[30]

EFFECTIVENESS OF PRE-HAB

Studies at Beth Israel Deaconess Medical Center and Harvard Medical School in Boston, Massachusetts found that knee- and hip-replacement surgery patients who participated in water- and land-based strength training, aerobic and flexibility exercises for six weeks prior to their surgeries reduced their odds of needing in-patient rehabilitation by 73%.

"Even in a fairly brief time period, exercise (before surgery) paid off for participants. Their level of function and pain stabilized prior to surgery, whereas those who did not exercise got worse. The benefits of exercise before surgery are very clear: The more you can do for yourself physically before surgery, the better off you will be," says Daniel Rooks, Ph.D., assistant professor of medicine at Harvard Medical School.[31]

Exercise can also assist in fending off atrophy and generate strength prior to surgery. Upper body and core strength may contribute to better stabilization, which is especially helpful if you happen to lose your balance and need to catch yourself. It may also help with using crutches or a walker. If you are having back surgery, strengthening core muscles support the back. (With all I've been through over the years, I have found core strength to be vital and invaluable.)

Simply, pre-hab gets patients back on their feet and achieve post-surgery milestones more quickly.

HOW DO YOU GET PRE-HAB?

Ask your doctor for pre-surgery exercise recommendations and/or a prescription for a physical therapy consultation. Physical therapists can supply you with a wide variety of exercises that can be done at home or at the gym.

THEN...

- **Verify pre-hab coverage with your insurance company**. Be aware, pre-hab visits may count toward your total physical therapy allowance. This is a worthwhile question to ask your insurance company so that you don't unknowingly use your allotted post-surgery physical therapy sessions all on pre-hab.
- **Partner with your physical therapist**. A custom pre-surgical exercise regimen tailored to you can help maintain and build muscle strength. (Read more about the benefits of exercise on pages 95-98.)
- **Perform the exercises as recommended** at home or at the gym, prior to surgery.
- **Take advantage of all remaining physical therapy sessions after surgery**. Physical therapy is an important part of healing and your post-surgical care.

PRE-HAB WORKS

A friend of mine in his 80s needed a hip replacement, but he had to wait three months. Rather than sit around, he kept his strength up by biking (on a three-wheeler) around his neighborhood and working with a physical therapist, weight training and strengthening. This combination paid off and, following surgery, he was up, moving around and out of pain more quickly than anticipated.

Prior to my back surgery I worked with a physical therapist for several months. Physical therapy helped manage my pain prior to surgery and was a great source of support and encouragement for me. Physical therapy also kept me strong, which I believe contributed to my springing back after surgery. My physical therapist told me that his clients who did pre-hab and were in better shape going into surgery had more positive post-surgical outlooks and bounced back faster than his patients who put in little to no pre-surgery effort.

Pre-Surgery Diet and Nutrition Suggestions

. . .

In order to prepare for surgery, heal, recover and once again thrive, your body will require extra nutrients: vitamins, minerals, protein, good carbohydrates found in vegetables and fruit and healing fats found in butter and natural oils. Eating well is paramount. The good news is that the same foods that are good to eat following surgery are also good for preparing the body for surgery. Refer back to pages 77-88 for information on eating and drinking to support healing and recovery.

Proper hydration—extra hydration—prior to and following surgery is also important for many reasons including the prevention of constipation which often accompanies surgery. (See pages 87-88 on the importance of hydration.)

CONSIDER A PRE-SURGICAL VITAMIN AND MINERAL REGIMEN FOR HEALING

Given that healing requires a great deal of energy obtained from nutrients, and most people don't consume enough nutrient-dense healthy foods, some people (including myself) find a pre-surgical vitamin routine can be supportive in preparing the body for the rigors of surgery and recovery. (See pages 89-91 on vitamins for healing and pages 199-201 for sample pre- and post-surgical vitamin, mineral and herb protocols.)

Stop or Reduce Potentially Harmful Substances

*The time before surgery is a good time to cut back on
any excessive or unhealthy habits.*

■ ■ ■

Alcohol

While small amounts beer and wine may have some health benefits, alcohol is also considered a drug. When preparing for surgery, warnings or precautions taken to minimize negative drug interactions should be implemented with respect to alcohol as well.

It has been shown that even moderate amounts of alcohol prior to surgery can weaken the immune system and slow recovery. The most common alcohol-related complications include: (1) postoperative infections, (2) cardiopulmonary complications, (3) impaired wound healing and (4) bleeding episodes (alcohol dilates blood vessels, which can lead to post-operative bleeding). Since alcohol has a dehydrating effect on the body, it can also contribute to or worsen constipation.

If you are alcohol-dependent, you may require special attention if, following surgery, you experience symptoms of withdrawal. If dependence information is known ahead of time, doctors can be prepared for any symptoms that may occur and assist you through them.

Smoking

This is the perfect time to quit, or at least cut back. Plain and simple: Patients who smoke get more infections[32] and sometimes require longer periods of time on a ventilator and supplemental oxygen after surgery. If you are unable to quit smoking entirely, even cutting back both prior to and following surgery is helpful for healing.

The most common complications related to smoking (cigarettes, cigars, marijuana or other substances) are: (1) delayed or impaired wound and tissue healing, (2) greater scarring, (3) wound infection, (4) cardiopulmonary complications[33] and (5) possible interference with the actions of certain medications.

RECREATIONAL DRUG USE

If you're having elective surgery, stop recreational drug use prior. This includes anything ingested, smoked or injected, either legal or illegal. Stopping is good for your health and is for your safety.

While drugs have traditionally been put into two categories, "legal" (prescribed by a physician) and "illegal" (obtained off the street), when preparing for surgery the real issue is not whether a substance is legal or illegal, but rather how its use could impact your surgery and recovery. Some drugs can alter the effectiveness of anesthesia or post-surgery pain medications, create drug interactions, or cause other complications during or after surgery. Many substances can also affect how the body metabolizes anesthesia and pain medication.

For example, opiates such as oxycodone have similar properties to other opiates such as heroin. Individuals who have been using opiates (of any kind) will likely have an increased tolerance to pain management drugs that contain opiates and may require higher doses to manage pain, hence the importance of full pre-op disclosure. Your doctor is not there to judge you on your recreational drug use, but rather is concerned with your safety. A doctor who knows your habits can better prepare and care for you.

Having said all that, the most widely used and widespread addictive substances on the market today are both legal: caffeine and sugar.

CAFFEINE

Since caffeine may affect blood pressure, it's recommended to cut back or discontinue products that contain caffeine (coffee, tea, soda, diet pills, etc.) a week prior to surgery. If you have a four-cup-a-day habit, you may want to slowly step it down and wean off to avoid possible headaches.

AVOID OR CUT BACK ON SUGAR

"Sugar is the 'most dangerous drug of our time' and is easy to obtain.
Just as with smoking labels, soft drinks and sweet products
should come with warning labels
that sugar is addictive and bad for health."
Paul van der Velpen, Head of Amsterdam's Health Service, Holland

Eating sugar and foods high in sugar, corn syrup and carbohydrates causes blood sugar to rise (blood sugar spike), followed by a corresponding increase in insulin output which then causes blood sugar to drop. This drop in blood sugar can drain energy and leave the body jittery, nervous, anxious, short-tempered, moody, blurry and confused. Avoiding this cycle before and after surgery supports the body as it heals.

DISCONTINUING CERTAIN PRESCRIPTION AND BLOOD-THINNING MEDICATIONS

Some prescription and over-the-counter medications can cause bleeding during or after surgery. These medications include anticoagulants such as aspirin, ibuprofen, Coumadin or Warfarin, among others, and should be avoided for a period before surgery, as advised by your doctor. Ask your doctor for a list of medications to stop prior to surgery.

DISCONTINUING CERTAIN VITAMINS, MINERALS AND HERBS

Some vitamins, minerals and herbs (including protein powders that may contain these ingredients), like any other medicine, may interact with anesthesia or other drugs administered during or following surgery. Complications can include bleeding, interference with other medications and increased blood pressure. Examples include: vitamin E, iron, fish oil, garlic, St. John's wort, dong quai, ginseng, feverfew, ginko biloba, ginger, licorice, Coenzyme Q_{10} and glucosamine, among others.[34] Again, it's best to check with your doctor and follow their instructions regarding discontinuing and re-starting products prior to and after surgery.[xxviii]

[xxviii] Note: Having said that, I personally have a belief that includes vitamins, minerals and herbs for health and well-being. If this describes you, it is up to you to do your own research around this issue. Consult with physicians who have experience in this area and then present your doctor or surgeon with your findings. Not all doctors and surgeons have extensive knowledge in every avenue of healing arts. Perhaps you are the patient who teaches their doctor something new.

2: AVOIDING SURPRISES—WHAT TO EXPECT RIGHT BEFORE AND RIGHT AFTER SURGERY

If you're like me, and do better with more information,
this is the chapter for you!

■ ■ ■

While being prepared can help alleviate some pre-surgery anxiety, knowing more specifically what to expect around the immediate surgery experience—especially the pre-op routine—may provide even greater peace of mind for some. This is true for me. I found that knowing in advance what would happen (and when)—being empowered with knowledge—reduced my pre-surgery anxiety, which I believe translated into ease, grace and a more positive all-round experience for me. With less information I tend to experience anxiety and resistance caused by fear of the unknown. *Knowing exactly what to expect at each stage greatly lessened my anxiety.*

The information and checklists on the following pages are intended to guide you through the days just before surgery, what to expect at the hospital or surgical center and what to be prepared for immediately after surgery.

SOME EXAMPLES

When I was 21 years old, I had open-heart surgery. Even though I knew I was in good hands medically, I was scared; it was a surreal experience. After checking in at the hospital, it would have been really helpful if someone had explained the full pre-op routine, procedures and schedule to me. (Had I thought of it, I should have asked, but I didn't know what I didn't know and it didn't occur to me.) More specifically, it would have been nice to know—in advance—that the evening before my surgery, two aides—complete strangers to me—were going to arrive unannounced and without context and shave my entire body from the neck down (arms, legs, pubic hair, etc.) in preparation for open-heart surgery and then paint me with an antiseptic.[xxix]

Another excellent example was shared with me by a friend who had cataract surgery. While she had taken the time to thoroughly educate herself on the procedure, she wished someone had prepared her with the knowledge that the pre-op routine (which took place while she was awake—only light sedatives are traditionally used for cataract surgery) included immobilizing her head, body and arms by securely strapping them down. Although stabilization makes sense—to be sure a patient doesn't move during this delicate procedure—not knowing this in advance added a great deal of unnecessary stress to her experience (even more so had she also been claustrophobic). Additionally, patients are awake and alert during cataract surgery (and can hear everything), but cannot move due to the restraints and cannot see because their face is covered by a sheet. Being awake, but having your face covered, can also be stressful and disorienting, especially if you're not prepared with that information beforehand, or again, are even the slightest bit claustrophobic. My friend also wished her doctor had clearly explained how long everything would take; no one mentioned the hour-long pre-op routine which added to the estimated 45 minute surgery. She was also not told that she may experience a headache following the procedure from having her head strapped down.

Being fully informed of pre-op routines in both these cases could have alleviated stress and anxiety caused by the unknown and unexpected. My recommendation: *Be persistent with your questions to avoid any surprises that could cause you to loose your center going into surgery*. For some—myself included—an inquiry such as, "Please walk me through *exactly* what's going to happen the day of surgery from the minute I walk through the door and complete my paperwork," might be helpful.

[xxix] An example of how things change: The pre-op routine for open-heart surgery is dramatically different today than in 1989, when I had open-heart surgery. Now, many hospitals simply have patients shower with an anti-bacterial soap the evening before surgery. Shaving is only employed if you happen to have a hairy chest. (Which, for the record, I do not.)

The Day Before Surgery

■ ■ ■

☐ **Confirm your arrival time at the hospital or surgical center**. They should call and give you this information. If not, call and confirm check-in time yourself.

☐ **You may receive a call from your anesthesiologist**. In some cases your anesthesiologist may call you the night before surgery to: (1) discuss which method they will be using on you, (2) go over any restrictions and (3) answer any lingering anesthesia-related questions you may have. Tell your anesthesiologist if you (or another family member) have experienced previous reactions to anesthesia. If your anesthesiologist doesn't call, not to worry, you will meet them after you check in and have been taken back to the surgical pre-op area. (See page 159 for information on anesthesia methods and page 160 for questions you may want to ask your anesthesiologist.)

☐ **Confirm the person staying overnight with you** *at the hospital*. If you will be staying overnight at the hospital and would feel more comfortable and relaxed having someone with you, honor this feeling and make arrangements.

☐ **Confirm your ride home**. Remember, you will be required to have a ride home following surgery. If your driver isn't going to be in the waiting room, give the name and phone number of your reliable driver to the receptionist at check in. Having your advocate pick you up is a good idea since you may want them to hear your surgical outcome from your doctor and take post-op notes on your behalf before heading home.

If you would feel more comfortable having someone physically in the waiting room while you are in surgery, speak up and ask someone. This is a valid feeling and a good job for your advocate. Additionally, having your advocate, family member or power of attorney present in the waiting room during surgery could be valuable should any decisions need to be made during the procedure, such as a change in the planned procedure or an emergency.

☐ **If you live alone, confirm the family member or friend who has agreed to stay overnight with you,** *once you are home*. This applies whether you're having out-patient surgery, or if you've been in the hospital and just discharged. It is **mandatory** this person stay for at least the first 24 hours you are back at home, preferably longer, if possible. This is for your safety! If it's not possible for someone to stay longer than the first 24 hours, arrange to have someone drop by—or call—on a regular schedule to check on you and handle tasks or needs that arise.

☐ **Follow any "night before surgery" pre-op instructions you may have been given**. Some people may have been given special pre-operative instructions to follow, such as using an antiseptic soap to wash with, special bowel prep, eye drops, etc. What's required will vary depending on the procedure and the hospital or surgical center's protocols; some pre-op instructions are more involved than others. For your safety, follow instructions carefully.

☐ **Shower and wash your hair the night before (or morning of) surgery**. It might be a few days before you are able to, or feel up to, showering or washing your hair following surgery. *After you shower, do not use any lotions, creams, powders, sprays, perfumes or deodorant* (even the night before). When you have surgery, your skin is being cut and broken into and your innards exposed, leaving it vulnerable. Even though the surgical site is thoroughly cleansed prior to making an incision, once the body is opened up, anything on your skin (even from another area) could get inside and cause a problem, such as an infection. It is easier, and safer for you, to avoid this possible complication altogether.

☐ **Do not shave, especially near the surgical site**. Shaving can irritate the skin or leave small cuts or abrasions which may leave the body vulnerable to infection.

☐ **Remove fingernail polish**. Some studies suggest fingernail polish can interfere with pulse oximeter readings. The pulse oximeter is a device used to monitor oxygen saturation in the body (see image on page 158). While there is ongoing research and debate as to whether or not nail polish really affects a pulse oximeter reading, I personally choose to err on the side of caution. If it's possible to get a more accurate reading without nail polish, then no nail polish for me. My health and safety are worth more than polished nails in the hospital.

☐ **Eat lightly—but well—the day before surgery**. Avoid heavy meals that can take a long time to digest. Loading up on greasy pizza or fast food the day or night before a surgery is NOT a good idea. Steamed fish or grilled chicken with steamed or grilled vegetables is a better choice.

☐ **Do not eat or drink anything after midnight or for at least ten hours prior to surgery**. No snacks or fluids (including no water). No sucking on candy; no nothing. This is for your safety. Anything in your stomach during surgery can lead to complications. The primary concern is that general anesthesia can cause nausea and vomiting. If a patient vomits while under anesthesia there is a risk the vomit could be aspirated into the lungs which can be dangerous or, in worst-case scenarios, fatal. Vomiting or stomach reactions can also interfere with the anesthesiologist's equipment or the surgery itself.

Ultimately, restrictions on eating before surgery are precautionary measures; emergency surgery may be performed on a patient who has recently ingested food or liquid. However, for scheduled procedures, eating and drinking before surgery should be avoided. If you do end up drinking or eating before surgery, for any reason, tell your anesthesiologist and surgeon.

☐ **If you start to feel sick or get a fever, call your surgeon**. If you are ill, your surgery may need to be postponed. Your surgery will have the best outcome if you are healthy when it begins.

☐ **Fill post-op prescriptions**. If possible, prefill prescriptions prior to surgery so they are at home when you return. Note: Some prescriptions may fall into a category of medications/drugs called Controlled Substances, which require a hard copy prescription (they cannot be phoned in by the doctor) and a photo I.D. to be picked up. Controlled Substances[xxx] include: (1) pain medications such as oxycodone (Oxycontin, Percocet), morphine, hydromorphone (Dilaudid), meperidine (Demerol) or codeine; (2) steroids (such as testosterone) and (3) sleeping pills such as benzodiazepine drugs (Xanax, Alprazolam, Clonazepam, Klonopin, Diazepam, Valium, Lorazepam).[35]

☐ **Pack for an overnight (or extended) hospital stay**, if necessary. While the hospital will provide essentials (soap, shampoo, etc.), you may be happier with your own products. (See packing list ideas on page 154.)

☐ **Confirm child or pet care arrangements**.

☐ **Water your plants**, indoors and outdoors.

☐ **Relax**. You have done all you can do and are in expert hands. Take a nap; the extra rest will do you good!

[xxx] A full list of all Controlled Substances can be found on the U.S. Department of Justice Drug Enforcement Agency Office of Diversion Control website at DEADIVERSION.USDOJ.GOV/SCHEDULES/INDEX.HTML.

Hospital Overnight Bag Checklist

NOTE: ITEMS 1-7 ARE ESSENTIAL; THE OTHERS ARE OPTIONAL.

- ☐ 1. **Insurance card**
- ☐ 2. **Personal identification**, such as a driver license or passport
- ☐ 3. **Personal medical file/notebook/journal/medical information**
- ☐ 4. **Current list of prescription and over-the-counter medications, vitamins, minerals and herbs** you are taking, the strength, dose and frequency.[xxxi] (Use the templates on pages 180 and 181 to help organize this information.)
- ☐ 5. **Glasses.** Glasses (vs. contact lenses) are recommended, as: (1) you will not be allowed to wear contact lenses into surgery and (2) contacts can become dry and uncomfortable if you are dehydrated or dozing after surgery.
- ☐ 6. **Inhaler medicine** (if you use it). To help with breathing, your anesthesiologist may ask you to take a dose just before surgery.
- ☐ 7. **CPAP machine.** If you have and use one, your doctor may have you bring it.

- ☐ **Reading glasses**
- ☐ **Cell phone and charger**
- ☐ **Earplugs** (and sleep mask, if you use one). Hospitals can be noisy, bright places.
- ☐ **Your pillow.** If you don't sleep well with a pillow other than your own, bring one from home. Label it with your name and phone number and put it in a bright pillowcase to differentiate it from hospital pillows.
- ☐ **Book, magazine, crossword or Sudoku puzzles, music, iPod, laptop computer** and earphones
- ☐ **Loose fitting clothes to wear home.** Make sure apparel will fit easily and comfortably over your incision and any brace (sweats, shorts, a button-up shirt, loose dress or skirt, slip-on shoes with good traction or flip-flops).
- ☐ **Cotton underwear.** (See page 28 for why cotton is a better choice.)
- ☐ **Toothbrush and toothpaste.** Include denture storage and cleaning kit, if necessary.
- ☐ **Hairbrush, shampoo, conditioner and soap.** If you prefer not to use what's provided by the hospital, bring your own.
- ☐ _____
- ☐ _____

[xxxi] Note: Some institutions may prefer you bring your actual daily prescription medications with you. Ask.

THE DAY OF SURGERY

．．．

☐ **Do not eat or drink anything the day of your surgery**. This includes not sucking on candy or mints or chewing gum. Sucking on candy or chewing gum increase fluids in the stomach—the stomach thinks food is coming and gets ready to receive it, which could add to the risk of anesthesia. If you have a medication that cannot be skipped, and it has been confirmed by your doctor that you should continue taking it, take it with a small sip of water and mention this to your nurse and anesthesiologist when you check in for surgery.

☐ **If you brush your teeth, do not swallow**.

☐ **Do not put on make-up**. Make-up is known to carry bacteria and even though the surgical site will be thoroughly cleansed it is easiest to avoid this potential complication by not wearing any at all.

☐ **Remove and leave all jewelry at home**. Wedding rings, necklaces, earrings, nose rings, belly rings, toe rings, watches, etc. Anything worn to a hospital or surgical center will have to be removed prior to surgery and will be safer at home.

☐ **Leave cash and credit cards at home**. Again, anything you take with you will be left behind and vulnerable once you change into your surgical gown and go into surgery. (If you are staying overnight, valuables will also be vulnerable while you are sleeping.)

☐ **Bring copies of consent forms and your Advance Health Care Directive**, if you have one.

☐ **Wear glasses if required to see**. Do not wear contacts; they will have to be removed.

☐ **Dress in comfortable, loose-fitting clothing**. Tight-fitting clothes may rub a tender incision, be hard to get back on or interfere with casting or bracing.

☐ **Mark your surgical site**. Everyone has heard horror stories or rumors of doctors operating on the wrong limb—the right shoulder instead of the left shoulder, for example. Protect yourself. Advising you to mark your surgical site is not to scare you, but rather to empower you and to avoid any confusion or miscommunication at the hospital

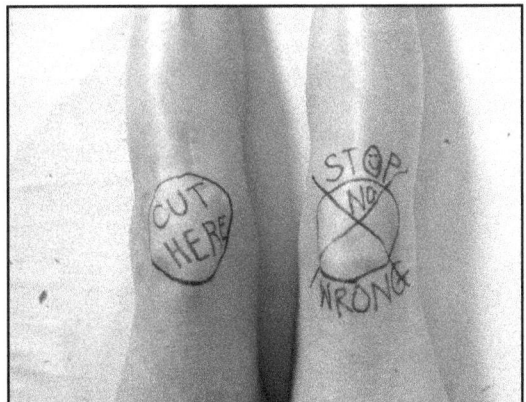

or surgical center. Take the initiative and clearly identify your surgical site. Doctors should ask you to do this, but in the event they don't, taking initiative and clearly marking your surgical site is good self-care—it is for your safety. Don't worry about offending your surgeon; they should appreciate you doing this. (Note: Some institutions prefer you *only* mark the surgical site, leaving the non-surgical site blank. Check beforehand. If no information is provided, do what will give you peace of mind.)

For those concerned that marker ink may introduce bacteria into an incision, there are many schools of thought on this. I'd personally prefer to mark my surgical site and avoid the wrong-site or wrong-side surgery. Some think that due to its alcohol base, a *single-use* Sharpie pen may be the safest to use. If you're concerned, do some research and decide what is best for you.

☐ **Arrive at the hospital or surgery center as directed**. This is typically one to two hours prior to surgery.

Keep breathing, you've totally got this!

WHAT TO EXPECT AT THE HOSPITAL OR SURGICAL CENTER

. . .

With approximately 11,000 hospitals and surgical centers in the U.S.,[36,37] each with slightly different routines, the following is intended to provide some broad stroke information on what to expect the day of your surgery. If having more specific or exact information would put you more at ease, ask someone at the hospital or surgical center to explain what to expect beforehand. If you're visually oriented and have time before your procedure, ask to tour the facility so you have a visual image and understanding of the process prior to check-in.

ARRIVAL

When you arrive at the hospital or surgical center you will need to present your identification and insurance card and will then be required to fill out and sign registration and surgical consent forms. Bring your complete list of medications, vitamins, minerals and herbs that you are currently taking. (See templates on pages 180 and 181.) If you're feeling anxious or nervous, remember to breathe.

After the paperwork is complete, and you're waiting to go back to the pre-op area, take a moment and close your eyes. Surround yourself, your doctors and the operating room in warm, white light. Ask your higher power for support. Take a few slow, deep breaths. This will help slow your heart rate and calm your mind. Any anxious feelings you may experience are normal, but remember, you are prepared. You've asked all the right questions, gotten organized and assembled a great team.

AFTER CHECK-IN

Once checked in, you will be escorted back to the pre-op surgical area where you will be given a surgical gown, cap and booties to change into and a bag to hold your clothes and any other items you have with you (insurance card, identification, dentures, hearing aids, wigs, hairpins, artificial limbs, etc.). Mark the bag with your name and phone number and give it to the nurse. If you are having an out-patient procedure, a nurse or nurse's aide will assist you with getting your street clothes back on following surgery. Otherwise, your belongings will be placed in your hospital room closet when you are moved from recovery to your hospital room. This is also your last chance to use the bathroom before surgery.

You will then be taken to the surgical area where you will get on a bed. At this time a nurse will begin the process of preparing you for surgery. A band will be placed on your wrist that includes your full name, birthdate and other pertinent information. Verify the information on the band is correct and remind the nurse if you have any allergies. If you have allergies, you may be given a second bracelet intended to alert doctors and nurses of your condition. The nurse will also hook you up to various monitors for your safety, including:

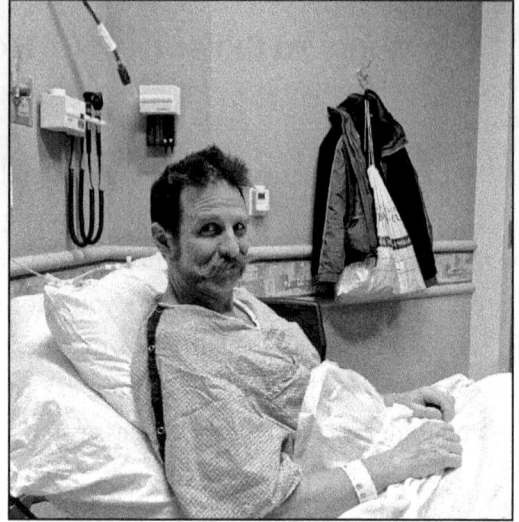
"Before." Prepared and relaxed.
(His advocate is in the waiting room.)

- **Pulse oximeter**. This clips on the end of a finger and measures your blood oxygen level.
- **Heart monitor**. Electrocardiography leads may be placed on your chest to record your heart rate and rhythm.
- **Blood pressure machine**. A blood pressure cuff will be placed on one arm to monitor the blood pressure in your arteries and heart.

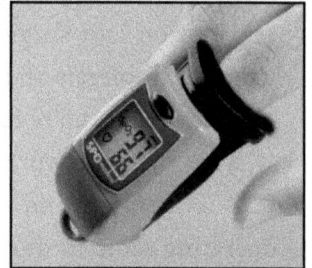
Pulse Oximeter

- **Other monitors?** This will vary based on the surgery you are having.

YOU WILL BE VISITED BY YOUR ANESTHESIOLOGIST

During this preparatory time, your anesthesiologist will stop by and review the anesthesia method being used on you and insert an intravenous tube (or IV) in the best vein on your arm or hand. You will receive anesthesia (and other) medications through this IV.

If you are feeling anxious—which is understandable and normal—communicate this. Your anesthesiologist can administer some medication to help you relax. It is not helpful for you to suffer. In fact, it is better if you are calm and relaxed (as much as possible) prior to going into the operating room.

Following preparations you will be taken to the operating room where anesthesia will be administered and the procedure performed.

Anesthesia Methods

Anesthesia is a medication used to prevent the feeling of pain, relax muscles and in certain cases induce temporary amnesia. There are three primary methods of anesthesia used to induce sleep and control pain during surgery. The method and medication used will depend on the type of operation you are having and your medical history.

Primary anesthesia methods: (1) general, (2) regional and (3) local, used with or without sedatives

(1) **General anesthesia**: Your entire body is "asleep" for surgery. This usually occurs in two stages. First, you will receive a drug through your IV that will make you drift off to sleep. The second stage of general anesthesia keeps you asleep during your surgery and can be administered through your IV or as a gas through a mask. If gas anesthesia is administered, a mask will be placed over your nose and mouth while you are still awake. With children, sometimes they are given gas anesthesia first and the IV line is inserted while they are asleep. General anesthesia may cause nausea following surgery. If you have previously experienced anesthesia-related nausea, let your anesthesiologist know before surgery.

(2) **Regional anesthesia**: Areas of the body are numbed so that you feel no pain. Common types of regional anesthesia are epidural, spinal and caudal anesthesia, which can numb large areas of your body, from your abdomen to your feet. Or, you may receive what is called a peripheral nerve block, which numbs smaller areas of your body. Little to no discomfort during surgery is reported by most patients who receive regional anesthesia. Regional anesthesia allows you to remain aware and observe your procedure, if you like. You may also receive other drugs with regional anesthesia that will make you drowsy or keep you in a light sleep.

(3) **Local anesthesia**: You may be awake and aware during the procedure or you may be given a medicine that makes you drowsy or puts you in a light or "twilight" sleep. Local anesthesia is often the preferred choice for minor surgical procedures or surgical injections such as a spinal epidural for pain management.

Whichever type of anesthesia you have, the anesthesiologist will monitor your blood pressure, pulse and breathing throughout the surgery or procedure and acute recovery period, until you are awake, alert, breathing on your own and ready to be discharged or moved to a non-surgical intensive care unit (SICU) hospital room.

QUESTIONS FOR YOUR ANESTHESIOLOGIST

ABOUT ANESTHESIA

- ☐ What type of anesthesia will I be given?
- ☐ What are the risks?
- ☐ Do I have a choice of which type of anesthesia I can get (general, regional or local)?
- ☐ What do you recommend? Why?

INFORMATION YOU SHOULD COMMUNICATE TO THE ANESTHESIOLOGIST:

- ☐ Previous anesthesia experiences (such as waking during surgery) or other reactions you, or any family member, may have had
- ☐ Personal anesthesia preference
- ☐ Past drug reactions
- ☐ Allergies
- ☐ Smoking history
- ☐ Medical and surgical history
- ☐ Dental information. Let the anesthesiologist know if you have any loose teeth, caps or crowns.

IMMEDIATELY AFTER SURGERY—THE RECOVERY ROOM

• • •

After surgery you will be taken to a recovery room, post-anesthesia care unit (PACU) or, if necessary, to a SICU where you will recover from the anesthesia. During this recovery period doctors and nurses will monitor your vitals and pain level as you awaken from surgery. Once awake and your heart rate, breathing rate and blood pressure are within acceptable limits, you will be moved to your hospital room or discharged if you had an out-patient procedure.

DEPENDING ON YOUR SURGERY, YOU MAY WAKE UP ON, OR WITH:

- **A ventilator**. This is when a breathing tube is in your throat, helping you breathe. If you awake with this still inserted, it will be removed once doctors see you are breathing successfully on your own.
- **Drainage tubes near the surgical site**. For example, when I awoke after open-heart surgery, there were three drainage tubes in my abdomen which were removed once I was fully stable and awake.
- **A small tube, or catheter, in your bladder**. This helps you urinate and makes it possible for doctors to monitor urine output which

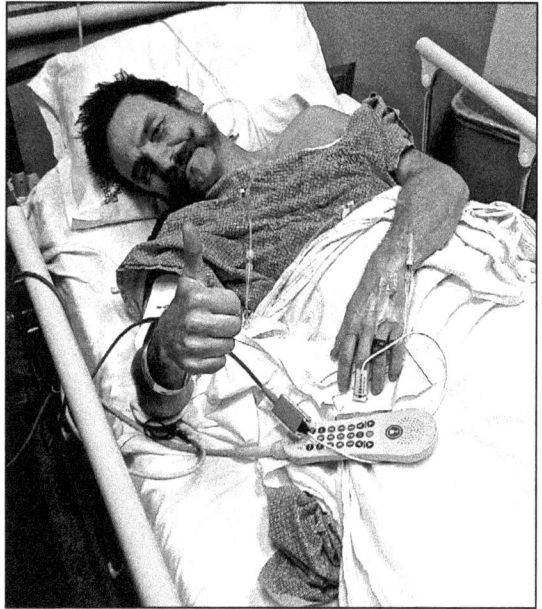

"After." Thumbs up. The face of success!

  provides them with information on how your bladder and kidneys are working. Catheters are easily removed after your doctor gives the all clear.
- **An IV**. The IV inserted prior to surgery will remain in place for the duration of your post-op care. Fluids and medications will be administered through your IV. A nurse will remove it prior to your release.
- **On oxygen**. You may wake up with tubing in both nostrils, wrapped around your ears. This tubing is used to deliver supplemental oxygen. Extra oxygen is to help with breathing and healing. It may tickle or itch, but leave it in place.

WHILE IN RECOVERY, TELL YOUR DOCTOR OR NURSE IF YOU EXPERIENCE:

- **Pain**
- **Nausea**
- **Dizziness**
- **A sore throat**

PAIN MANAGEMENT

*Controlling your pain after surgery is
an important part of your post-operative care and recovery.*

As you recover, your doctor will order pain medication for you based on your condition and pain level. The nursing staff is there to administer pain medication and assist with pain management throughout your stay. During your recovery, you will see more of the nurses than your doctor, so be sure to communicate with both your doctor and the nurses about your level of pain.

Since only you can assess your level of pain, you will be asked to rate your pain on a scale of 0 to 10 (0=no pain and 10=worst pain possible) both before and after each pain intervention. (Refer to Wong-Baker FACES illustration on page 62.) This provides valuable feedback on the effectiveness of the pain treatment and will assist your doctor in adopting a plan of pain management care that is appropriate for you.

Again, be sure to clearly communicate with your doctor and nurses about your level of pain so they can keep you comfortable. Suffering through unrelieved pain may do more harm than good.

BENEFITS OF PAIN CONTROL INCLUDE:

- **Greater comfort, including decreased stress and anxiety** caused by pain
- **Ability to walk, breathe more deeply and gain strength back** more quickly

BE SURE TO REPORT:

- **Unrelieved pain**
- **Any sudden onset of severe pain**
- **Side effects from pain medication**, which may include nausea, vomiting, itching, an inability to urinate, sleepiness, hallucinations, numbness or weakness in your legs, constipation. (See full list of pain medication side effects on page 64.)

NAUSEA AND DIZZINESS

Nausea and dizziness are common side effects associated with anesthesia. They can also be caused by pain or pain management medications you have been given. Depending on your situation, your doctor may, or may not, prescribe medication to relieve these discomforts (such as an anti-nausea medication). If your doctor does prescribe something, it will likely be administered through your IV.

WHY DOES MY THROAT HURT?

Your throat may hurt after surgery for two reasons: (1) you may be dehydrated, since you haven't had anything to eat or drink since the night before surgery or (2) your throat may be irritated from the intubation process. If a breathing tube is required during surgery, it will be inserted after you are asleep. A tube is placed in your mouth, down the throat and then attached to a ventilator to help you breathe. This process can irritate the vocal cords. This tube is often removed before a patient regains consciousness, sometimes leaving them to wonder why their throat is sore. Care of any residual sore throat should include resting vocal cords and drinking lots of fluids. If your sore throat lasts longer than a week, consult your surgeon or doctor.

YOUR ROLE IN RECOVERY

...

DEPENDING ON YOUR PARTICULAR SURGERY, INSTRUCTIONS MAY VARY, BUT WILL LIKELY INCLUDE:

☐ **Get moving!** When possible and advised, walk early and walk often. Depending on the procedure you have undergone, you may be prompted (even pushed) by the nurse to get moving fairly quickly. Patients with better mobility will be released sooner. There are many benefits to moving and walking after surgery including: helping blood flow return to normal, preventing the formation of blood clots, preventing pneumonia (walking helps move bacteria-infested mucus out of the lungs), reactivating the peristaltic movement (contractions) in the bowels, relieving gas and preventing constipation.

☐ **Deep breathing and coughing**. To help prevent fluids from building up in the lungs, which can lead to pneumonia or other dangerous infections, your doctor or a nurse may ask you to breathe deeply and cough. You may also be given a device called an incentive spirometer which measures deep breaths and keeps your lungs in shape. Deep breathing using the device will help you get better faster.

☐ **Use the bathroom**. Prior to being released from either a hospital or surgical center you will be required to urinate and in many cases, especially following major surgery, have a bowel movement.

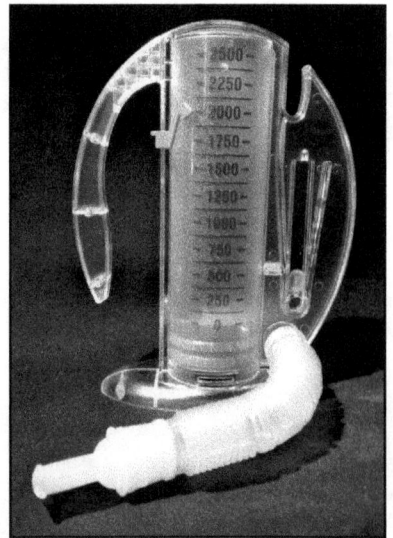

Incentive Spirometer

These functions, successfully performed, indicate your bladder is awake and working and there is no bowel obstruction. Urinating is important because if the bladder fills up completely and is not relieved, fluid can back up and can cause damage to the bladder and kidneys.

The inability to urinate after surgery is usually caused by a neurogenic bladder, which basically means that the nerves of the bladder aren't communicating with the brain, so in spite of discomfort or pain, the bladder continues to fill and in extreme cases can rupture.

General anesthesia puts the entire body to sleep, including the bladder and abdominal muscles, and it can take time for everything to wake up. A delay in urinating can be caused by the physical trauma of surgery, anesthesia, anxiety and pain (or other) medications given during or after surgery. Once you urinate, it becomes easier and easier to do so because you are flushing anesthesia and other medications out of your system.

If you have a history that includes difficulties urinating, bring this to the attention of your doctor before surgery. For patients with no history or difficulty urinating prior to surgery, any difficulty after surgery should completely resolve with time.

POST-SURGERY GOALS

The goal of post-surgery care is to help you become independent so you can be discharged and return home. When you are discharged, you should be able to:

- ☐ **Get in and out of bed** by yourself
- ☐ **Safely walk the hallway**, with or without a walker
- ☐ **Climb stairs**, if needed at home
- ☐ **Use the bathroom**, including toileting and bathing or showering
- ☐ **Be able to eat and drink on your own**
- ☐ **Care for your incision**
- ☐ **Understand recovery instructions**

BEFORE YOU GO HOME

• • •

Once it's determined you're ready to be discharged from the hospital or surgical center, a nurse will assist you in getting your street clothes on and you will receive instructions from your doctor on continuing your recovery at home. Since you may be fuzzy from anesthesia or pain medication, have someone (your advocate or a family member) ready with a pen and paper to take notes; they can go over instructions with you once you are home and settled. Make sure everyone is clear on post-op surgical instructions such as administering or applying medications and changing bandages or dressings. Get a demonstration so you can see it being done properly. *Important: Have a solid discharge plan that you feel safe and comfortable with in place **before** going home. Ask as many questions as you need. Be sure you **get an after hours phone number** where you can reach a doctor with any questions or concerns.*

This is also the time to request a complete copy of all your hospital medical records so you can take them with you when you leave; you will want them for your files and it can be harder to get them after the fact.

YOUR RECORDS SHOULD INCLUDE:

- ☐ Discharge summaries—why you were admitted and your discharge diagnosis
- ☐ Pathology reports
- ☐ CT and MRI scans, x-rays and reports
- ☐ Surgical reports
- ☐ Progress notes
- ☐ Emergency room records

WHEN YOU ARE DISCHARGED, YOU SHOULD ALSO RECEIVE:

- ☐ Incision or wound care instructions (including bathing and showering instructions)
- ☐ Activity instructions
- ☐ Special diet instructions, if necessary
- ☐ Instructions for any medications you are to continue (dosage, time and frequency)
- ☐ Follow up appointment instructions for your surgeon or other doctors
- ☐ Instructions on what to do and who to call if an emergency, or other questions arise after you get home.

IMPORTANT TIP ABOUT EMERGENCIES OR QUESTIONS THAT ARISE AFTER YOU ARE DISCHARGED AND BACK HOME

Be sure to get a phone number you can call after hours or on weekends should an emergency or other question(s) arise outside normal doctor office hours. Without this information, should an emergency or other question arise after doctors have left the office for the evening or weekend, the only recourse is to wait until the next business day or to take a patient to an emergency room.

I ran into this scenario after my 86-year-old father had shoulder surgery. Back at home he had problems with nausea and vomiting. Due to this complication, he couldn't keep down medication, food or fluids and he started to become weaker. Even though it was outside of normal business hours, in an effort to reach a doctor for advise, I called his surgeon's office, thinking there would be someone on-call. Instead, the answering machine said, "If this is an emergency, call 911." I wasn't ready to do that, but still very much wanted to speak with a doctor about my questions and concerns.

My next call was to the hospital where my father's surgery was performed. This became a frustrating experience because no one would answer my questions; they just keep transferring me. They told me that since my father was no longer an in-patient, no one was able to advise me or help me. Worst of all, no one was willing to call my father's surgeon or the surgeon's physician assistant and have them call me. Furthermore they said that even if they wanted to help, they were unable to verify that I was who I said I was on the phone (his daughter and his medical power of attorney), so they could not give me any information. Each person I spoke with just said to take him to the emergency room. While I remained calm (trying the approach that you get more bees with honey than vinegar), I couldn't understand from my perspective why no one was able to put me in touch with a doctor who could help. I felt scared and abandoned by the medical community.

The good news is, *you can avoid this experience by getting an after hours phone number that a patient—or their advocate or caregiver—can call with any questions or concerns that may arise once back at home!*[xxxii]

[xxxii] On the positive side, some surgical facilities do provide an after hours contact number as part of their discharge plan. This was the case for another family member (who had surgery in a different state). When he was discharged from a same-day surgical center the nurse gave him and his wife a number to call where a doctor would be available 24/7 to assist them with questions, big or small. The nurse even highlighted this important information on the discharge papers.

QUESTIONS TO GET ANSWERED BEFORE HEADING HOME

☐ **How did the surgery go?** Did you find anything unusual or unexpected?

☐ **Is there anything I should be aware of or expect at home** (such as drainage from the incision or blood in my stool, for example)?

☐ **Medication information**: Knowing how to correctly take prescribed medications and administer or apply prescribed eye drops, eye ointments, oral rinses or wound creams, is important.

    ☐ When/what time of day?

    ☐ How much?

    ☐ How often?

    ☐ Are there any side effects?

☐ **Incision care**: (See pages 40-41 for more on incision care.)

    ☐ What do I need to know about my incision?

    ☐ Any special instructions? Things to do, or not do?

    ☐ When do I get my stitches out?

☐ **What are the signs of infection?** (See pages 44-47 for more on the signs of infection and other complications following surgery.)

☐ **What number should I call if I have questions or concerns outside of normal business hours?** (After 5:00P, on the weekend or on holidays.)

☐ **When should I follow up with the doctor and/or surgeon?** If possible, schedule this appointment before going home. (See page 114 for more on post-surgical follow up.)

☐ **When should I begin physical therapy?** (See pages 92-93 for more on physical therapy after surgery.)

☐ **When can I shower or bathe?** (See pages 42-43 for more on showering and bathing after surgery.)

☐ **What about physical activity?** Do I have any limitations? If yes, what? For how long?

☐ **When is it safe to drive?** (See pages 132-133 for more on driving after surgery.)

☐ **When can sexual activities be resumed?** (See pages 99-100 for more on sex after surgery.)

☐ **When can I return to work or school?**

A Final Word

Remember at the beginning when I said, "you don't know what you don't know"? Here's what I've learned and know for sure:

We need support!
And we also need love, compassion, encouragement,
fresh air, sunshine, enough sleep, exercise, good food and water!

■ ■ ■

While experts—doctors, nurses and therapists—are there to help and support you before, during and after surgery, *you are in charge or your successful surgery and healing.* Follow instructions and don't be afraid to ask questions. Most important is you; your safety, your comfort and your recovery.

Here's to your successful surgery and healing!

RESOURCES:

SAMPLE TEMPLATES AND APPENDIX

SAMPLE TEMPLATES

The templates[xxxiii] on the following pages are designed to help you generate and organize information. Having this information prepared ahead of time will keep you from feeling overwhelmed and potentially frustrated when nurses and doctors ask what may feel like an endless barrage of questions. Do you take any medications? How much? How often? For what? Have you ever had surgery before? When? Why? And so forth.

Once you've collected and organized this information, save it in a special file or on your computer so it's available if you need it in the future. Update this file as you go. Having this information prepared can be particularly helpful when seeing a new doctor or in the event of an emergency.

MEDICAL AND HOSPITALIZATION HISTORY

For your medical and hospitalization history, include everything you can remember. If you can't remember, ask family members and friends if they can help you remember.

[xxxiii] All of the templates included on pages 176-186 and 190-191 are also available as free .DOCX and .PDF downloads at LORIMERTZ.COM.

One reason for a detailed medical history is so that your doctor is aware of any previous injuries or surgeries you've had that may be relevant to your current surgery. For example, prior surgeries, in a close proximity, may have slightly rearranged things in that area or left some residual scar tissue. This may also provide important information about any negative reactions you have had. For example, reactions to antiseptic solutions, tape, anesthesia or any medications.

For hospitalizations, include anything that required you to be admitted to a hospital, such as an illness, injury or surgery and the dates. Include the outcome and any complications or reactions to treatments. The more detail, the better. (Use template on page 177.)

HERE ARE SOME EXAMPLES OF ITEMS TO INCLUDE:

- Tonsillectomy (age, date)
- Fractured right arm from fall on playground (date)
- Allergies such as cat fur, pollen, shellfish, nuts, eggs, latex, medications (such as lidocaine, penicillin, etc.). Include diagnosed age, date, if you received allergy shots, etc.
- Appendectomy (age, date)
- Car accident (age, date, injuries)
- Hip replacement (age, date)
- Diagnosed with autoimmune condition (age, date)
- Colonoscopy (age, date and results)
- Pneumonia (age, date and action—did it require hospitalization?)
- Pregnancy (age, number of pregnancies and births and the dates)
- Other conditions, disease diagnoses, orthopedic injuries or surgeries

DAILY PROGRESS LOG

With a progress log you can chart your progress and look back and see all the milestones you've hit. It will let you see when, where and how you are improving. This log is especially helpful if you feel like you aren't progressing or getting better, which can be frustrating.

This tool was particularly helpful for me following unrelenting headaches and pain from my head injury. My doctor recommended making notes on everything about my headaches including how bad they were, what kind of pain I was experiencing (sharp, dull, throbbing, etc.), where in my head I felt the pain, if the headache moved around, how long the headache lasted, if anything made it better or worse, what medication I took to help and how well it worked, what I ate and drank, every detail; again, the more information, the better. It helped my doctor help me.

When I found myself struggling, referring back to my notes and seeing that, even though I might be having a bad day or week, I was in fact getting better overall, was encouraging. Seeing where and when my pain decreased from a nine to an eight to a six to a three was huge. Being able to see my progress, such as a day or two between headaches and then a week and then a month between headaches, for example, was exciting. Healing was a day-by-day, minute-by-minute process that, in this particular case, took years, but it did take place. I got better. (Use template on page 183.)

EMERGENCY CONTACT INFORMATION

It can be handy to have all important phone numbers in one place. Having doctor and provider phone numbers together can create a great resource for you, your family or your advocate in the event of an emergency. Be sure to include and clearly delineate your health care power of attorney. (Use template on pages 178-179. Additionally, see pages 188-199 which outline documents recognized in the event of an emergency.)

TEMPLATES:

- ☐ **Patient Information**, page 176
- ☐ **Medical History & Hospitalizations**, page 177
- ☐ **Emergency Contact Information**, pages 178-179
- ☐ **Current Medications**, page 180
- ☐ **Current Vitamins, Minerals and Herbs**, page 181
- ☐ **Doctor Appointment Notes**, page 182
- ☐ **Daily Progress Log**, page 183
- ☐ **Pain Management Rating Scale and Tracking Calendar**, page 184
- ☐ **Monthly Calendar (blank)**, page 185
- ☐ **People Who Have Offered to Help**, page 186

PATIENT INFORMATION

BLOOD TYPE, ALLERGIES, INTOLERANCES AND SENSITIVITIES

(Protected health information. Keep in a secure place.)

■ ■ ■

PATIENT INFORMATION:

Name:_____   Date of birth:_____

Address:_____   Place of birth:_____

_____

Phone/cell:_____

Email:_____

BLOOD TYPE (FOR DONOR PURPOSES):

(NOTE: LIST FAMILY OR FRIENDS WITH COMPATIBLE BLOOD TYPES WHO LIVE NEARBY (WHO HAVE NOT HAD ILLNESSES THAT PRECLUDE DONATING.))

Patient's blood type:_____

Donor name/relation:_____   Donor name/relation:_____

Donor name/relation:_____   Donor name/relation:_____

ALLERGIES, INTOLERANCES AND SENSITIVITIES:

(I.E., LACTOSE INTOLERANT OR CAFFEINE SENSITIVE. INCLUDE DRUG, FOOD AND ENVIRONMENTAL CAUSES.)

Allergies:_____

_____

_____

Intolerances:_____

_____

_____

Sensitivities:_____

_____

_____

MEDICAL HISTORY AND HOSPITALIZATIONS

(Protected health information. Keep in a secure place.)

■ ■ ■

PATIENT:_____

PATIENT MEDICAL HISTORY:
(INCLUDE EVERYTHING: SURGERIES, INJURIES, ILLNESSES, ETC.)

Date:_____

Issue/diagnosis:_____

Notes:_____

Date:_____

Issue/diagnosis:_____

Notes:_____

Date:_____

Issue/diagnosis:_____

Notes:_____

Date:_____

Issue/diagnosis:_____

Notes:_____

Date:_____

Issue/diagnosis:_____

Notes:_____

Date:_____

Issue/diagnosis:_____

Notes:_____

EMERGENCY CONTACT INFORMATION

. . .

PATIENT:_____

Surgeon name: _____

Surgeon phone: _____

Surgeon office address: _____

Hospital name: _____

Hospital phone: _____

Hospital address: _____

Internist name: _____

Internist phone:_____

Internist office address: _____

Other doctor name: _____

Other doctor phone:_____

Other doctor office address: _____

NOTE: CLEARLY DELINEATE PATIENT'S MEDICAL PROXY, IN THE EVENT OF AN EMERGENCY.

Primary emergency contact:

Name:_____

Phone: _____

Secondary emergency contact:

Name:_____

Phone: _____

Relative, friend, neighbor, other:

Name:_____

Phone: _____

Name:_____

Phone: _____

Name:_____

Phone: _____

Name:_____

Phone: _____

Name:_____

Phone: _____

Name:_____

Phone: _____

Name:_____

Phone: _____

CURRENT MEDICATIONS
PRESCRIPTION OR OVER-THE-COUNTER—TAKEN FOR ANY REASON

(Protected health information. Keep in a secure place.)

■ ■ ■

PATIENT:_____

A/O (current date):_____

MEDICATION (BRAND/GENERIC NAME)	STRENGTH & DOSAGE	REASON	FREQUENCY

CURRENT VITAMINS, MINERALS AND HERBS

TAKEN FOR ANY REASON

(Protected health information. Keep in a secure place.)

■ ■ ■

PATIENT:_____

A/O (current date):_____

VITAMIN/MINERAL/HERB	STRENGTH & DOSAGE	REASON	FREQUENCY

DOCTOR APPOINTMENT NOTES

• • •

Doctor's name: _____   Date of visit: _____

Doctor's phone: _____   Things to take: <u>Notebook, pen, voice recorder, other</u>

Question: _____

_____

Response: _____

_____

_____

_____

Question: _____

_____

Response: _____

_____

_____

_____

Question: _____

_____

Response: _____

_____

_____

DAILY PROGRESS LOG

. . .

PATIENT:_____

LIST ANY CHANGES, NOTES OR UPDATES (ON PAIN, SYMPTOMS, MEDICATIONS, DIET, REACTIONS, ETC.) OR OTHER THINGS YOU NOTICE:

Date:_____

Progress notes:_____

_____

_____

_____

Date:_____

Progress notes:_____

_____

_____

_____

Date:_____

Progress notes:_____

_____

_____

_____

Date:_____

Progress notes:_____

_____

_____

_____

PAIN MANAGEMENT SCALE AND TRACKING GUIDE

■ ■ ■

PAIN MANAGEMENT RATING SCALE AND TRACKING CALENDAR

Patient: _____   Date: _____

Wong-Baker FACES® Pain Rating Scale

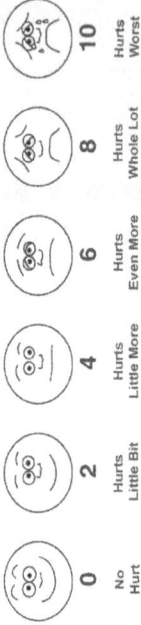

0	2	4	6	8	10
No Hurt	Hurts Little Bit	Hurts Little More	Hurts Even More	Hurts Whole Lot	Hurts Worst

©1983 Wong-Baker FACES® Foundation. Visit us at www.wongbakerFACES.org. Used with permission. Originally published in Whaley & Wong's Nursing Care of Infants and Children. ©Elsevier Inc.

Tips:
- Choose the face that best depicts the pain you are experiencing (see Wong-Baker FACES Pain Rating Scale to the right).
- Make notes about your pain levels and on the pain intervention taken (what you did or what medication you took) and its effectiveness.
- Take time to notice daily and weekly improvements (even small ones), they add up.

DATE	TIME	PAIN RATING	PAIN INTERVENTION TAKEN (Medication or supplement and dosage and/or other technique such as meditation or exercise.)	SIDE EFFECT(S)	EFFECTIVENESS

Successful Surgery and Healing, lorimertz.com, 052715

MONTHLY CALENDAR
(To do's, appointments, notes, things to remember, etc.)

■ ■ ■

MONTHLY CALENDAR

_____ , 20 _____ (Year)
(Month)

SUNDAY	MONDAY	TUESDAY	WEDNESDAY	THURSDAY	FRIDAY	SATURDAY
(Date)						

NOTES or EMERGENCY CONTACTS:

Successful Surgery and Healing, lorimertz.com, 05271⁵

People Who Have Offered To Help

· · ·

WHO/PHONE/EMAIL	WHEN/AVAILABILITY	WHAT (Driving, meals, errands, etc.)

APPENDIX

Documents Recognized in the Event of An Emergency

• • •

A Special Power of Attorney and Living Will are documents that should be kept with your will and other important legal documents and should be updated periodically, should the need to use them ever arise.

Health Care Power of Attorney or Special Power of Attorney (SPOA)

These legal documents allow you to appoint another person (called an attorney-in-fact, agent or health care proxy) to make decisions for you, should you become temporarily or permanently unable to make decisions yourself. This will legally empower them to access your medical records, discuss your care with doctors and help make decisions. It allows someone to respond to unanticipated health care situations. By appointing an agent, you can make sure health care providers abide by your wishes. Hospitals, doctors and other health care providers must follow your agent's decisions as if they were your own. You may give an agent as little or as much authority as you want. This form can also be used to document wishes or instructions on organ or tissue donation.[38] There are some good boilerplate resources for generating a SPOA available online with easy to follow step-by-step instructions, or you can have an attorney prepare one for you. The two online resources I found to be helpful were: (1) AMERICANBAR.ORG[39] and (2) STATE.IL.US, "Illinois Statutory Short Form Power of Attorney For Heath Care."[40] Laws can differ by state. Verify regulations for legal health care documents. Make sure copies of any legal documents are given to the appropriate parties, such as your health care proxy, doctor, spouse, advocate, lawyer or trusted friend.

Living Will

A living will deals with medical issues while you are living; it is different from a regular will or trust, which addresses distribution of assets after death. A living will tells your doctor whether or not you want life-sustaining treatments (which would only prolong dying) or procedures (such as mechanical respirators) administered if you are in a terminal or persistent vegetative state. If someone consents to be your health care proxy, it is important they understand that they have agreed to ensure and follow the stipulations listed in your Living Will. (See sample of a living will from the New York State Bar Association on pages 190-191.)

Note: Since undergoing surgery is a life-sustaining life-supporting procedure, a surgical patient with a living will that contains a "do not resuscitate" (DNR) order may need to reconsider and temporarily suspend this directive to undergo surgery. This is an important topic to discuss with your surgeon prior to surgery.

MEDICAL TREATMENT PLAN

A medical treatment plan is created by you and your doctor after you have suffered an injury or before an operation or medical procedure that may result in impairment or death. Your doctor will generate this plan and review it with you prior to surgery or any other treatment.

SAMPLE LIVING WILL

(New York Living Will—NYSBA.ORG)

■ ■ ■

I, _____, being of sound mind, make this statement as a directive to be followed if I become permanently unable to participate in decisions regarding my Medical care. These instructions reflect my firm and settled commitment to decline medical treatment under the circumstances indicated below.

I direct my attending physician and other medical personnel to withhold or withdraw treatment that serves only to prolong the process of my dying, if I should be in an incurable or irreversible mental or physical condition with no reasonable expectation of recovery.

These instructions apply if I am: a) in a terminal condition; b) permanently unconscious; or c) if I am conscious but have irreversible brain damage and will never regain the ability to make decisions and express my wishes.

I direct that treatment be limited to measures to keep me comfortable and to relieve pain, including any pain that might occur by withholding or withdrawing treatment. While I understand that I am not legally required to be specific about future treatments, if I am in the condition(s) described above, I feel especially strong about the following forms of treatment.

I do/do not want cardiac resuscitation.

I do/do not want mechanical respiration.

I do/do not want tube feeding.

I do/do not want antibiotics.

I do/do not want maximum pain relief.

Other instructions (insert personal instructions):

I HEREBY APPOINT

Name: _____

Address: _____

_____

Phone Number: _____

as my health care agent to make all health care decisions for me in conformity with the guidelines I have expressed in this document. I direct my agent to make health care decisions in accordance with my wishes and instructions as stated above or as otherwise known to him or her. I also direct my agent to abide by any limitations on his or her authority as stated above or as otherwise known to him or her.

In the event my health care agent is unable, unwilling, or unavailable to serve as such, **then I appoint as my substitute health care agent** (with the same powers that I have heretofore enumerated).

Name: _____

Address: _____

_____

Phone Number: _____

I understand that unless I revoke it, this living will and health care proxy will remain in effect indefinitely. These directions express my legal right to refuse treatment, under the laws of the state of _____. Unless I have revoked this instrument or otherwise clearly and explicitly indicated that I have changed my mind, it is my unequivocal intent that my instructions as set forth in this document be faithfully carried out.

Signature: _____

Address: _____

_____

Date: _____

Statement By Witnesses (Must Be 18 or Older)

I declare that the person who signed this document is personally known to me and appears to be of sound mind and acting of his or her own free will. He or she signed (or asked another to sign for him or her) this document in my presence.

Witness: _____

Address: _____

Witness: _____

Address: _____

KEEP THIS SIGNED ORIGINAL WITH YOUR PERSONAL PAPERS AT HOME. GIVE COPIES OF THE SIGNED ORIGINAL TO YOUR DOCTOR, FAMILY, LAWYER AND OTHERS WHO MIGHT BE INVOLVED IN YOUR CARE.

More About Massage Therapy and Bodywork

▪ ▪ ▪

Finding the right massage therapist and receiving the right bodywork for you

The type of surgery you have will determine when you can begin receiving bodywork and what modalities may serve you best. Choosing the right form of bodywork (modality) for your situation can make a difference in how you feel and how quickly you heal after surgery.

It's important the therapist you go to is licensed. Education and experience are essential. To locate a good massage therapist in your area, ask your physical therapist or a trusted friend or call a local massage school for recommendations of a licensed massage therapist who specializes in injury and recovery and has a medical focus.

I have used the modalities described below with positive results. My body responds well to healing touch, but moreover, I believe the kindness, compassion and support I received from the wonderful practitioners I was fortunate to find and work with also played a valuable role in my healing and recovery.

The following is a sampling of techniques that may be helpful with pain management and healing after surgery.

Light Touch Massage

Light massage can be soothing and relaxing prior to or following surgery, allowing the body to function more optimally during the healing process. A light touch massage may be appropriate soon after surgery, assisting blood and lymph flow and gently soothing aching muscles. This type of massage can help you to relax and release tension, calm the nervous system and aid rest and sleep.

Reflexology

Reflexology is also an excellent form of bodywork to have in the first days or weeks after surgery; it has no contra-indications (unless you had surgery on your feet), soothes the central nervous system and is highly relaxing. Reflexology allows the therapist to address all of the systems of the body through the feet. It is so safe and effective it's used on infants and children who are in the hospital.

Lymphatic Drainage Therapy

Lymphatic drainage therapy is also a light touch modality; it assists the healing process by promoting lymph flow and lymph node function.

The lymph system is at the forefront of the body's immune system and comes in contact with every cell in the body. Lymph fluid cleanses tissues and removes toxins, debris and damaged or dead cells that are the result of trauma from injury or surgery. Unlike the circulatory system, the lymph system does not have a pump helping it circulate throughout the body. Instead, the contractions of our muscles keep lymph moving and valves in the lymph vessels keep the fluid from flowing backwards. When a person is confined to bed for a period of time, due to illness, injury, or recovery from surgery, the lymph can become sluggish, which may result in edema, slowed healing and a less efficient immune system. Additionally, incisions, the formation of scar tissue and the removal of lymph nodes may block lymphatic pathways.

Receiving lymph work can help in healing the surgery site and with scar tissue that is forming at this time. A lymphatic drainage therapist can help to redirect the lymph, relieve edema and promote healing. Lymphatic drainage therapy also has a positive effect on the parasympathetic nervous system that aids relaxation.

CRANIOSACRAL THERAPY

Craniosacral therapy is a gentle hands-on method that deals with the cranial sacral rhythm/system in the spine, including the bones of the head, spinal column, sacrum and the underlying structures. Craniosacral therapy removes restrictions around the spinal cord and taps into the inherent wisdom of the body, allowing it to heal itself. It is an incredibly gentle, restorative therapy that alleviates headaches and stiffness and eases pain, leaving the body feeling light, relaxed, calm and peaceful.

DEEP TISSUE MASSAGE

As you progress in your recovery, your massage therapist could recommend deep tissue work. Deep tissue massage can break up knots in the muscles, including trigger points that may have formed. It can also reduce scar tissue adhesions and help break up any scar tissue that may have formed. This work requires the therapist to have a solid background in anatomy.

FELDENKRAIS METHOD

The Feldenkrais Method allows the body to move and function more efficiently and comfortably by re-educating the nervous system and improving motor ability. This is very subtle, slow, gentle work, which is widely recognized and often used by physical therapists. Many physical therapy clinics now have Feldenkrais practitioners on staff.

I am grateful to have worked with a long-time Feldenkrais practitioner. Through our work I experienced profound results including ease of movement, significant pain reduction and greater mobility. The work translated even further to include improved posture, greater stability on my feet, better overall balance and an expanded understanding of my brain-body connection. I was thrilled as I effortlessly went from painful situations, to having no pain and regaining full range of motion.

ESSENTIAL OILS

Long venerated for their healing properties, essential oils can be used to facilitate relaxation or conjure and stimulate happier feelings. The right combination of essential oils can promote relaxation and relieve feelings of anxiety and stress before, or after, surgery. They can be used by themselves or added to massage oil.

Essential oils of basil, bergamot, chamomile, clary sage, geranium, jasmine, lavender, melissa, neroli, patchouli, rose, sandalwood and ylang ylang can assist in relieving depression and rosemary, peppermint, lemon, basil, ginger, tea tree and cypress can stimulate and awaken your system.[41]

Lavender and chamomile together, in particular, have tremendous relaxation properties, as well as anti-bacterial and anti-microbial properties. When I want to rest, they really do the trick. I've used this mixture in my bath, in a candle and mixed with some grapeseed oil, massaged into my skin; it's very soothing.

More About Energy Work

■ ■ ■

Reiki

Reiki is an ancient Japanese healing energy technique for stress reduction and relaxation that also promotes healing. Reiki is a simple, gentle, non-physical, natural and safe method that works in conjunction with any medical or therapeutic technique to assist and promote healing.

Cardio-thoracic surgeon Mehmet Oz, M.D. has used Reiki and other energy techniques to balance patients' energy during open-heart and heart transplant surgeries.[42,43] One research study showed that patients who received Reiki had significantly improved sleep (by 86%), reduced pain (by 78%), reduced nausea (80%) and reduced anxiety (up to 94%).[44]

I have received Reiki and been grateful to experience similar results when healing from the traumatic effects of surgery.

Therapeutic Touch

Therapeutic Touch is an evidenced-based, holistic therapy that incorporates the intentional and compassionate use of universal energy to promote balance and well-being. It is a non-invasive, easily accessible healing modality, based on the premise that human beings are comprised of energy and we are more than our physical body.[45]

Today, over 50 thousand nurses are trained in Therapeutic Touch in the U.S.[46] and it is practiced in major hospitals across the United States, Canada and around the world.[47] If you are an in-patient at a hospital, ask if they have someone certified in Therapeutic Touch on staff.

Crystalline Consciousness Technique

Crystalline Consciousness Technique (CCT) is an energy technique that helps release shock and pain from the body while accelerating healing. CCT also helps transform and release underlying energy patterns that may have been present before surgery.

While a newer energy technique, the value of CCT has been recognized by nurses and is accredited by the American Holistic Nurses Association for continuing education credits.

CCT helped me find stillness and recalibrate my energy after my head trauma.

Meditation and Relaxation Exercises

■ ■ ■

Meditation can be as simple as sitting or lying quietly, with your eyes relaxed or closed and breathing slowly and steadily through your nose. As you breathe, let thoughts drift away. If they return, or your mind wanders, gently refocus attention on your breathing.

Since the mind can only really focus one thing at a time, if you're focused on your breath, it cannot be thinking thoughts. If you find it helpful, add some soft instrumental or meditation music and focus on that. Try sitting still for just five to ten minutes and see how you feel.

Relaxation—good anytime, anywhere

I have found that checking in with my body and taking short breaks throughout the day can be helpful in relieving tension and keeping pain at bay. Here is one quick easy relaxation sequence that can be done anywhere, anytime.

- Begin by noticing what's going on around you. Then interrupt and switch your thoughts to yourself and your breathing. Sit up, take a few deep breaths and exhale slowly.
- Mentally scan your body. Notice areas that feel tense or cramped, such as your neck or shoulders. Breathe and allow your shoulders to drop. Let go of as much as you can.
- Slowly rotate your head to the left in a smooth, circular motion, leaning your left ear to your left shoulder. Rotate your head to the right in a smooth, circular motion, leaning your right ear to your right shoulder. (Stop any movements that cause pain.)
- Roll your shoulders up and down, forward and backward several times. Notice tension releasing and falling away. Allow your muscles to relax.
- Smile. A simple smile relaxes facial and cranial muscles. It can also activate the release of the feel-good neurotransmitters dopamine, endorphins and serotonin that fight off stress and even lower heart rate and blood pressure.[48] Recalling and focusing on a pleasant memory can have a similar effect.
- Take another deep breath and exhale slowly. *Ahhhh.*

Progressive muscle relaxation—great for sleeping

Progressive muscle relaxation involves sequentially tensing and then relaxing muscle groups in the body, one at a time. The key to this exercise is to tighten a specific muscle group for three to five seconds, until you feel the tension, and then release the muscles. Notice the difference in how the muscles feel before and after.

- Start by getting into a comfortable position in bed.
- Beginning at your feet, slowly moving toward your head, tense and release each muscle group, one at a time, avoiding the surgical site. Toes, feet, ankles, calves, knees, thighs, gluts, abdomen, hands, arms, chest, shoulders, neck, jaw, ears, face, scalp. Tighten and relax. Tighten. Relax.

This exercise is wonderful for several reasons: (1) it forces the mind into the present moment, (2) the comparison of tensing and relaxing muscles provides the body with information on what relaxation really feels like and (3) it is good for unmasking hidden areas of tension. Perceiving one extreme (tightening) allows for the experience of feeling the other extreme (relaxation). When I have trouble sleeping, I use this exercise. I have never made it more than half way before falling asleep. Try it.

VISUALIZATION EXERCISES

• • •

Find a quiet spot. Begin by knowing that your doctors and their staff are collaborating with you for healing, health and wholeness. Everyone and everything is working for you.

Then, use your mind to visualize your unique recovery process; a graceful, successful, supported surgery and recovery. What does it look like for you? What do you see yourself getting back to doing? In addition to visualization, add in your feelings, 'feelization.' How does it feel? Include all your senses and emotions.

For some, creating a story can help.

EXAMPLE 1

Imagine your body as a town that has been hit by a hurricane (surgery). Now notice the townspeople cautiously emerging from their homes, coming out and coming together to partner and rebuild. It's a community effort. Your body is made of a community of cells (50 trillion cells, give or take) that work together and cooperate with one another. Hold a town meeting to discuss the details. If you're experiencing swelling in an area, imagine the community coming together and breaking down a dam in that area, so blood pools can disperse. If you want to experience blood flow to an area, imagine them cooperating in such a way that a pathway, tunnel or bridge is built, so blood can get to and access an area. If you want your bones to mend and heal, use the image and feeling of a Gothic cathedral, solid and built to withstand the test of time. If you have a low white blood cell count from an infection, use the imagery of a dragon slayer, slaying and eradicating all invasive species from your body temple.

EXAMPLE 2

Imagine your body is the garden and you are there tending to it; feeding and watering it, fertilizing it with nutrients and vitamins, gently pulling and eliminating any weeds. Imagine your garden so vibrant and healthy that it can withstand any attack from bugs, weeds, germs or other unwanted invaders. Imagine how the soil feels and how it smells, its richness. Notice the sweet fragrance of the flowers. Feel the warmth of the sun on your skin and soft breeze on your face. Hear the wind rustling through the trees and the buzz of a hummingbird whizzing by. Gently weed out any unwanted plant species. Carefully dig and remove the entire body and root of a weed. Add some rich, nutrient-dense compost and carefully refill the hole. Experience growth, strength, nurturing, healing and delight on all levels in your garden as it grows and thrives.

Sample Vitamin, Mineral and Herb Regimen For Healing

∎ ∎ ∎

The following information has been very helpful for me personally. In the context of this book, it is informational only for those interested in further supporting and complementing other prescribed treatments. As noted earlier, there are instances where supplementation may be contraindicated. It is up to each individual to decide what is right for them and to communicate that to their doctor so a safe doctor-supported plan can get generated. I am particularly lucky because my doctor is well-schooled and well-versed in supplementation for healing, health and well-being. Building on pages 89-91, Dr. Mangum recommends the following for two to four weeks prior to surgery (if possible) and four to six weeks after surgery.

Prior to surgery:

- **Multivitamin/mineral**: Choose a high-quality, high-potency, full-spectrum vitamin. (See a few of my favorite brands on page 204.)

In addition to the multivitamin/mineral also include the following:

- **Vitamin C**: Vitamin C enhances and strengthens immune system function, fights off infection and promotes healing. It is an important factor in collagen production, which promotes tissue healing and recovery from surgical wounds.
- **Bioflavonoids**: Bioflavonoids work together with vitamin C, increasing the uptake of vitamin C and maximizing its benefits. In general, flavonoids are useful as antioxidants, antivirals and anti-inflammatories and pack a punch against free radicals. Flavonoids are found in bright and dark vegetables and fruits and not in synthetic, pre-packaged convenience foods or fast foods.
- **Zinc**: Zinc supports healthy cell growth and immune system function, among other properties.
- **Copper**: Copper works with iron to form healthy red blood cells. Copper also helps to produce energy in cells, form a protective covering of your nerves and connective tissues, maintain the health of your bones and connective tissues, help keep your thyroid gland functioning normally and reduce tissue damage caused by free radicals.
- **Vitamin A**: Vitamin A is a fat-soluble vitamin important for the immune system, supporting organs (heart, lungs, kidneys) in functioning properly and is a precursor to active hormones.
- **Vitamin E/Mixed Topherols**: Vitamin E is a fat-soluble vitamin with strong antioxidant properties, which means it can help protect human tissue, cells and organs.
- **Vitamin D3**: Also known as the sunshine vitamin, vitamin D3 has many benefits including protecting against insomnia and depression.

FOLLOWING SURGERY ALSO INCLUDE:

- **Pancreatin** or **Bromelain**: Pancreatin and bromelain are known for their digestive and anti-inflammatory properties.

IF YOU ARE TAKING AN ANTIBIOTIC ALSO ADD:

- **Saccharomyces boulardii**: For those on antibiotics following surgery (or struggling with digestive issues), replenishing healthy intestinal microflora is important. Microflora are a major regulator of the immune system in the gut and other organs. Antibiotics can disturb the balance of yeast in the intestines and kill friendly bacteria, leaving intestines vulnerable to "bad" bacteria and yeast overgrowth. Saccharomyces boulardii is beneficial yeast that antibiotics won't kill. It is also used to help prevent and treat diarrhea caused by the use of antibiotics.[49] The Langone Medical Center's Department of Surgery recommends continuing with Saccharomyces boulardii for two weeks after the last dose of antibiotics is taken to restore natural digestive tract bacteria.

  Saccharomyces boulardii is found in the refrigeration section at health food stores.

OTHER HELPFUL VITAMINS AND SUPPLEMENTS:

- **B Vitamins**: Taking B12 during the day can aid in a good night's sleep, play a role in melatonin production, ease stress, promote a healthy immune system, support metabolism of carbohydrates and fats, boost energy and improve mood and memory. B vitamins are also critical to circulation and adrenal hormone production. They also boost the immune system and support a healthy mood and feelings of well-being.
- **Fish oil**: Fish oil has many great properties. A large and growing body of scientific evidence indicates that fish oil supports internal repair systems that operate in response to physical stress and injury, circulation, lung function, healthy blood vessel function, healthy brain function and positive moods. Fish oil has also been shown to improve and maintain digestive and gastrointestinal health; promote a healthy immune response; contribute to joint health, including, flexibility, mobility and comfort; protect against free radicals; and enhance endurance and recovery.

  In choosing a good fish oil, be sure the product has been assayed for purity (third party tested and approved) and is free of heavy metals and PCBs (polychlorinated biphenyl, a group of toxic industrial compounds, which have been outlawed for decades).[xxxiv]

[xxxiv] Note: Cod liver oil has been shown to contain high levels of PCBs. Avoid shark oil as well—top predators live for long periods of time and are known for being high in mercury. Fish, like sardines, with short lifespans are better because they don't have time to eat or absorb lots of toxins.

In the end, no amount of vitamins can replace the most important things we need: nutritious fresh food and clean water, deep sleep and exercise. These are the foundation of our health.

TWO RECIPES I CAN'T LIVE WITHOUT

. . .

I couldn't resist sharing my two of my favorite recipes that are easy, quick, delicious and nutritious. In addition to their health benefits, both the chia and hemp seed porridge and smoothies contain ingredients helpful for combating constipation.

CHIA AND HEMP SEED PORRIDGE

Place 2 tablespoons of chia seed and 2 tablespoons of hemp seed in a bowl. Add 1 cup of boiling water. Stir briefly and let it sit for approximately three minutes. (Use more or less water to adjust mix to desired thickness. I like it a little more moist so add slightly more boiling water.)

Then add some of your favorite fresh fruit (I use peaches, raspberries, blueberries and tangerines depending on what is in season) and top with some organic plain yogurt (I like goat milk yogurt) or coconut milk. Stir it up and voilà, a delicious healthy meal.

You can also add other nutrient-rich stir-ins such as goji berries, golden berries (both known as superfoods), shredded coconut, cashew pieces, a little coconut milk (which adds healthy fat) and more. (I have had it with some vanilla whey protein powder stirred in as well, which adds more protein and a little sweetness.)

PROTEIN SMOOTHIE

In a blender combine:

1-2 scoops of protein powder as per directions on container (I prefer vanilla whey protein)

1 cup frozen fruit (I use frozen organic berries)

1/4 can (2-4 oz.) of coconut milk (use regular coconut milk—avoid "light" coconut milk which is the same price, but contains less good fat, which is partly what you're eating it for)

1-2 T fish oil (I like Nordic Naturals which contains natural lemon flavor and tastes great)

1 cup water (more or less—depends on how thick you prefer it)

You can also add other nutritious ingredients—experiment!:

- Chia seed
- Hemp seed
- Ground flaxseed
- Fresh ginger
- Green or superfood powder
- Plain whole yogurt (try goat's milk yogurt)
- Avocado (Yes, avocado. It sounds crazy, but it adds good fat and vitamins and makes it extra creamy. Try it.)
- Pineapple (including the core, which is a good source of the anti-inflammatory enzyme bromelain)

Blend it up and voilà, healthy protein snack and energy boost!

Recommended Reading, Websites and Resources

The following resources have provided both insight and inspiration for me through their powerful and profound words, teachings and support.[xxxv]

■ ■ ■

Surgery and health-related reading and resources

Bailey, Elizabeth, *The Patient's Checklist*, Sterling Publishing, 2011

Balch, Phyllis A., CNC, *Prescription for Nutritional Healing, Fifth Edition: A Practical A-to-Z Reference to Drug-Free Remedies Using Vitamins, Minerals, Herbs & Food Supplements*, Avery Penguin Group Publishing, 2010

Calton, Ph.D., Jayson and Calton, CN, Mira, *Rich Food Poor Food: The Ultimate Grocery Purchasing System*, Primal Blueprint Publishing, 2013

Caring Bridge, Free online support calendar for coordinating care, meals, posting updates and other support, CARINGBRIDGE.ORG

Chopra, M.D., Deepak, *Quantum Healing: Exploring the Frontiers of Mind Body Medicine*, Bantam Books, 1989

Christensen, Tiffany, *Sick Girl Speaks!*, iUniverse, 2007

Cousins, Norman, *Anatomy of an Illness As Perceived by the Patient: Reflections on Healing and Regeneration*, W. W. Norton & Company, Inc., 1979

Curtiss, Karen, *Safe and Sound in the Hospital: Must-Have Checklists and Tools For Your Loved One's Care*, Partner Health LLC, 2012

Hay, Louise L., *You Can Heal Your Life*, Hay House Inc., 2004, HAYHOUSE.COM

Lipton, Ph.D., Bruce, *The Biology of Belief: Unleashing the Power of Consciousness, Matter and Miracles*, Mountain of Love/Elite Books, 2005

Mangum, M.D., Todd, Web of Life Wellness Center, WEBOFLIFEWC.COM

[xxxv] For additional recommendations see *Resources* at LORIMERTZ.COM/RESOURCES.HTML.

National Institute On Aging, *Talking With Your Doctor: A Guide For Older People*, National Institutes of Health, 2005

Roizen, M.D., Michael F. and Oz, M.D., Mehmet C., *You The Smart Patient: An Insider's Handbook for Getting the Best Treatment*, Free Press, 2006

Siegel, M.D., Bernie S., *Love, Medicine & Miracles: Lessons Learned About Self-Healing from a Surgeon's Experiences with Exceptional Patients*, Harper Row, 1986

University Pharmacy, UNIVERSITYPHARMACY.COM

Weil, M.D., Andrew, *Spontaneous Healing: How To Discover and Embrace Your Body's Natural Ability to Maintain and Heal Itself*, Random House Publishing Group, 1995

■ ■ ■

SOME FAVORITE BRANDS

The following products are available at your local health food store, through their websites, via online retailers such as AMAZON.COM, or through health care providers as noted.

Allergy Research*, ALLERGYRESEARCHGROUP.COM

Designs For Health*, DESIGNSFORHEALTH.COM

Jarrow Formulas, JARROW.COM

Natural Vitality, NATURALVITALITY.COM

Nordic Naturals, NORDICNATURALS.COM

PURE Encapsulations*, PUREENCAPSULATIONS.COM

Rainbow Light, RAINBOWLIGHT.COM

The Synergy Company, THESYNERGYCOMPANY.COM

Thorne Research*, THORNE.COM

Trace Minerals, TRACEMINERALS.COM

---

* Some brands are only available through professional health care providers.

Index

FDA. *See* U.S. Food and Drug Administration
Feldenkrais, 193
fever, 45
feverfew, 148
fiber, 55
    insoluble, 55
    soluble, 55
    supplements, 56
fish oil, 87, 148, 200
FMLA. *See* Family Medical Leave Act
fresh air, 21, 97, 110
frostbite, 49
garlic, 148
gastrocolic reflex, 57
gastrointestinal, 52, 53
Gaudet, M.D., Tracy, 107
genetically modified (organism), 81
GI. *See* gastrointestional
ginger, 148
ginko biloba, 148
ginseng, 125, 148
glucosamine, 148
gluten-free, 31
GMO. *See* genetically modified organism
goals, 76, 92
gratitude, 109
handicap parking, 133
Happy, 111
Harvard Medical School, 113, 143
head injury, 174
headache, 47
health care proxy, 188
heart monitor, 158
hemp seed, 84, 202
hospital bed, 140
hospital food, 84
Huddleston, Peggy, 113
HULU.COM, 22
hydration, 50, 54, 87–88
hypertension, 58
hypnosis. *See* hypnotherapy
hypnotherapy, 70
hysterectomy, 134
I'm Alive, 111
ibuprofen, 48, 49, 50, 63, 125, 131, 148
ice, 48, 65
incision care, 39–43
infection, 131, 146
infection, signs and symptoms
    fever, 45
    hardening, 44
    hot, 45
    incision opens, 46

malise, 45
    numbness, 44
    pain, 45
    pus, 44
    red streaks, 44
    redness, 44
    swelling, 44
inflammation, 48–50
insomnia, 110, 199
insulin, 86, 96
insurance, 74, 132, 134, 138–39
    pre-authorization, 138
    questions to ask, 120, 134, 137, 140, 141
iron, 148
Jarrow Formulas, 204
Katie, Byron, 110
Krazy Glue, 40
lab work, 126
label reading, 81
lactose intolerant, 31
Langone Medical Center, 200
lavender, 194
laxatives, 53, 56
    herbal, 56
legal documents
    Living Will, 137, 188, 190–91
    Medical Treatment Plan, 137, 189
    Special Power of Attorney, 137, 188
licorice, 148
Lipton, Ph.D., Bruce, 108, 112
Living Will, 137, 188
    Sample Living Will, 190–91
long-arm grabber, 23
long-handle shoehorn, 23
Love, Medicine & Miracles, 107, 204
low blood sugar, 96
lymphatic drainage therapy, 192
macrophages, 48, 95
magnesium, 54–55
magnesium sulfate. *See* Epsom salt
make-up, 155
Mangum, M.D., Todd, 77, 78, 83, 199, 203, 211
Massachusetts General Hospital, 211
massage therapist, 192
massage therapy, 112, 192–94, 69–70
    craniosacral, 193
    deep tissue, 193
    essential oils, 194
    Feldenkrais, 193
    light touch, 192
    lymphatic drainage, 192
    reflexology, 192
    Therapeutic Touch, 195

Acknowledgements

Did you know that everything you've ever done
and everywhere you've ever been has brought you to
this moment, right here, right now?

■ ■ ■

Summing up acknowledgements is a tremendous challenge given the magnitude of experiences, influences and individuals that I believe contributed to and made this book possible and a reality.

The first major medical and surgical experience I had, in 1988, would set my bar for medical care and would shape all my experiences to follow: being diagnosed with Wolff-Parkinson-White syndrome (WPW) and subsequently having open-heart surgery.

To two of the kindest, gentlest, most heart-centered men, who happened to also be brilliant cardiologists and cardiothoracic surgeons, Brian McGovern, M.D. and Gus Vlahakes, M.D. at Massachusetts General Hospital; thank you from the bottom of my heart. It is a rare few who can tell someone how they've touched your heart and have it be true both literally and figuratively.

To neurosurgeon Sylvian Palmer, M.D., Rosemary Palmer, RN and their staff who many, many years later, showed me what a successful, fully supported surgery and recovery can look like. I was terrified to have back surgery, but in too much pain to live without having it. Dr. Palmer's infinite patience as he explained the problem and walked me through what to expect, in spite of my ever-present terror, was an awesome experience for me. I wish all doctors and their staff were as dedicated to their patients' physical, mental, emotional and spiritual well-being.

To Todd Mangum, M.D., whose care and integrative medicine practices have changed my life over the past 15-plus years. Thank you for being a doctor who listens and makes their patients partners in their health care. Thank you for the hours you spent consulting and helping me tweak the medical and nutritional portions of this project.

To Greta deJong and Alice Toler, my editors and dear friends. I wouldn't be here now had it not been for your encouragement, support, brilliance, wisdom, insights, patience, editing and teaching. Being an editor is a special job and you both do it with such grace and ease. How lucky I am to get to work with you. Thank you for your belief in me and this project and for reviving me as I neared the finish line. We need people to believe in us in order to succeed!

To my long-time friend and teacher, gia combs-ramirez, who is awesome at getting to the bottom of any conundrum in a minute or less and saying the right thing at the right time, especially when things feel the gloomiest.

To Chris Harding, who tirelessly answered questions and provided much needed business coaching and perspective along this epic journey.

To Michael Bernard Beckwith, founder of Agape International Spiritual Center, whose teachings have inspired me in countless ways and have been a power-full avenue of support and encouragement. "Life *is* good!" Thank you Rev. Michael. Thank you Rev. Greta, Rev. Kathleen, Rev. Cheryl, Rev. Leon, Akili and each member of the Agape International Spiritual Center Community. You guys got it right—we need each other! I am so grateful for all you have shared and taught me!

And to my family members and friends who have loved me, listened to me, encouraged, supported and walked my path with me through surgery, recovery and the writing and completion of this book—how blessed and grateful I am. Mom, thank you for being there in sickness and in health and being a constant cheerleader.

When someone believes in us, all things are possible.

Champions show up in our lives in a million different ways—big and small—and serve as inspiration when we need it most. How could I possibly include them *all*? And in what order? Ann, Bert, Betsy, Britnee, Carol, Chris, Dad, Debbie, Duane, Eric, Gilbert, Gina, Jane, Jason, John, Jon, Josh, Lesley, Lila, Lisa, Megan, Merle, Dr. Petron, Rebecca, Simon, Stacie, Steve, Sue, Terrie, Tony and Dr. Whitley.

I am continually inspired by the stories people have shared with me, and all I continue to learn. I am also continually reminded of how much we really need each other and how lucky I feel to be here now, where I have crossed paths with more incredible souls than I ever imagined.

And so it is, with a great and full heart that I release this material, embedded and sealed with the vibration of love, peace, wholeness, health and well-being. May it be of service to everyone who picks it up.

About the Author

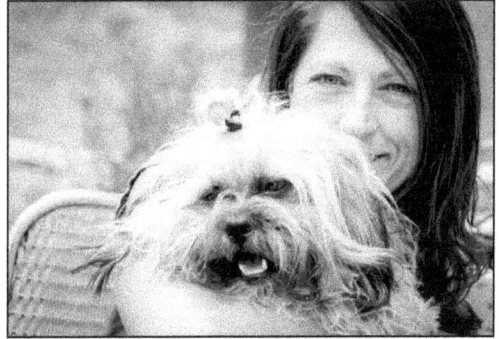

Born and raised in Southern California, Lori Mertz currently resides in Salt Lake City, Utah with her four-legged companion (and Zen-master) Engelbert Oscar Hummingbird aka 'Bert.'

Her studies and inquiring mind have taken her from Southern California to Arizona State University to Boston, Massachusetts to a classroom in the Shivagakomarpaj Traditional Medicine Hospital in Chiang Mai, Thailand, to the Himalaya in Nepal, to a 16-week journey across India and to Salt Lake City. For over 20 years Lori has worked in Utah as a production manager and production coordinator in the film and entertainment industry. She has also been a practicing licensed massage therapist since 2003 and a passionate life-long volunteer for many organizations including those that support foster children, the homeless, U.S. veterans, brain injury and disaster relief.

Lori's credentials and expertise also come from extensive personal field research from both planned and unplanned surgery including: a partially severed Achilles tendon, open-heart surgery, an emergency appendectomy, reconstructive knee surgery, a traumatic brain injury and back surgery. She has also worked as a patient advocate for family and friends and continues to learn and grow from ongoing conversations with doctors, nurses, physical therapists and patients.

With all she has learned from her studies, travels and her own surgical and healing experiences, Lori hopes the information and stories shared through her work will support and encourage others as they prepare for, undergo and recover from surgery, trauma or illness, back to their state of perfect health and wholeness. "I want to touch, move and inspire others as so many have done for me. If we are here on planet Earth on purpose, for a purpose, then with my life experiences, this is one of mine—sharing what I've learned to help, support and empower others going through similar experiences. Here's to paying forward all that my experiences, doctors, therapists and healers have taught me over the years."

For more information on Lori, her passions and projects, or to book her for coaching sessions, consulting or speaking engagements, visit: LORIMERTZ.COM, LORIMERTZ.BLOGSPOT.COM, FACEBOOK.COM/SURGERYANDRECOVERY.

You Are Your Own Temple.
Treat Yourself Accordingly.

Notes

[1] Gupta, Sanjay, "More Treatment, More Mistakes," *New York Times*, July 31, 2012, http://nytimes.com/2012/08/01/opinion/more-treatment-more-mistakes.html.

[2] Vespa, Jonathan, Lewis, Jamie M., and Kreider, Rose M., "America's Families and Living Arrangements: 2012," U.S. Census Bureau, censes.gov, http://www.census.gov/prod/2013pubs/p20-570.pdf, 1.

[3] Heisler, RN, Jennifer, "Know When Your Symptoms After Surgery Are an Emergency, *About.com*, August 14, 2011, http://surgery.about.com/od/aftersurgery/a/ERAfterSurgery.htm.

[4] Heisler, RN, Jennifer, "All About Constipation: What Exactly Does Constipation Mean?," *About.com*, February 26, 2011, http://surgery.about.com/od/aftersurgery/ss/ConstipationSur.htm.

[5] Ibid.

[6] Grant, BSc, Joshua A., Rainville, PhD, Pierre, "Pain Sensitivity and Analgesic Effects of Mindful States in Zen Meditators: A Cross-Sectional Study," *Psychosomatic Medicine Journal of Biobehavioral Medicine*, January 2009, vol. 71 no. 1, 106-114, http://www.psychosomaticmedicine.org/content/71/1/106.abstract.

[7] Orme-Johnson, PhD, David W., Schneider, M.D. Robert H., Young, Son D., Nidich, PhD, Sanford, Cho, PhD, Zang-Hee, "Neuroimaging of meditation's effect on brain reactivity to pain," January 2, 2008, http://www.ncbi.nlm.nih.gov/pmc/articles/PMC2170475.

[8] Marchand, M.D., William R., "Mindfulness-based stress reduction, mindfulness-based cognitive therapy, and Zen meditation for depression, anxiety, pain, and psychological distress," *Journal of Psychiatric Practice*, July 18, 2012, http://www.ncbi.nlm.nih.gov/pubmed/22805898.

[9] Cole, Adam, "Even Beginners Can Curb Pain With Meditation," *NPR.org*, April 6, 2011, http://www.npr.org/blogs/health/2011/04/08/135146672/even-beginners-can-curb-pain-with-meditation.

[10] "Meditation: An Introduction," National Center for Complementary and Alternative Medicine, National Institute of Health, June 2010, http://nccam.nih.gov/health/meditation/overview.htm.

[11] American Psychological Association, July 2, 2004, "Hypnosis for the Relief and Control of Pain," http://www.apa.org/research/action/hypnosis.aspx.

[12] Elkins, Gary, Jensen, Mark P., Patterson, David R., "Hypnotherapy for the Management of Chronic Pain," *International Journal of Clinical and Experimental Hypnosis*, Volume 55, Issue 3, 2007, http://www.ncbi.nlm.nih.gov/pmc/articles/PMC2752362.

[13] combs-ramirez, gia, "Do You Have One Ability You'd Never Give Up?," *Science of Energy Healing*, http://scienceofenergyhealing.com.

[14] Magee, MPH, RD, Elaine, "Fast-Food French Fried: Which Are Healthiest?," *WebMD.com*, March 18, 2009, http://www.webmd.com/food-recipes/features/fast-food-french-fries-which-are-healthiest.

[15] Reader's Digest, "4 Most Harmful Ingredients in Packaged Foods," *RD.com*, http://www.rd.com/health/diet-weight-loss/4-most-harmful-ingredients-in-packaged-foods.

[16] Cousins, Norman, *Anatomy of an Illness As Perceived by the Patient: Reflections on Healing and Regeneration*, (W. W. Norton & Company, Inc., 1979), 31.

[17] Baum, PhD, Andrew & Poluszny, PhD, Donna M., "Health Psychology: Mapping Bio-behavioral Contributions to Heath and Illness," *Annual Review of Psychology*, 1999, Vol. 50, 137-163.

[18] Aronson, MS, RD, Dina, "Cortisol—Its Role in Stress, Inflammation, and Indications for Diet Therapy," *Today's Dietitian*, November 2009, Vol. 11, No. 11, 38.

[19] Society for Endocrinology, "Cortisol," *You and Your Hormones*, September 5, 2012, http://www.yourhormones.info/hormones/cortisol.aspx.

[20] Schwartz, L.C.S.W., Mel, "Beyond the Mind-Body Connection," *A Shift of Mind*, January 23, 2010, http://www.psychologytoday.com/blog/shift-mind/201001/beyond-the-mind-body-connection.

[21] Salmansohn, Karen, *Instant Happy: 10-Second Attitude Makeovers*, Ten Speed Press Berkeley, 2012.

[22] Cousins, Norman, *The Healing Heart: Antidotes to Panic and Helplessness*, W. W. Norton & Company, 1983.

[23] Siegel, M.D., Bernie S., *Love, Medicine and Miracles: Lessons Learned About Self-Healing from a Surgeon's Experience with Exceptional Patients*, Harper & Row, Publishers, Inc., 1986, back cover.

[24] Lecture, Lipton, Ph.D., Bruce, July 21, 2013, Institute of Noetic Sciences 15th International Conference and 40th Anniversary, https://www.youtube.com/watch?v=NB09_LpXp90.

[25] Neibuhr, Reinhold, "The Serenity Prayer," 1943.

[26] Huddleston, Peggy, Book Description, http://www.amazon.com/Prepare-Surgery-Heal-Faster-Techniques/dp/0964575760.

[27] Lieblein, Virginia, Cohn, M.D., Lawrence H., Huddleston, Peggy, Interview, *Healthbeat* News, uploaded July 10, 2009, http://www.youtube.com/watch?feature=player_embedded&v=hQVs1vwietA#at=11.

[28] Schaub, M.D., PhD, Freidemann, "Accelerated Healing, Change and Self-Empowerment Through Mind-Body-Spirit Integration," *Cellularwisdom.com*, http://www.cellularwisdom.com/body-mind-healing.shtml.

[29] University of Maryland Medical Center, "Mind-Body Medicine," http://www.umm.edu/altmed/articles/mind-body-000355.htm.

[30] Rizzo, Terrie Heinrich, "Pre-hab for Surgery," *Arthritis Today Magazine*, Arthritis Foundation, 2009, http://www.arthritistoday.org/arthritis-treatment/surgery/preparing-for-surgery/prehab-for-surgery.php.

[31] Ibid.

[32] Stop Smoking for Safer Surgery, http://www.stopsmokingforsafersurgery.ca.

[33] Heisler, RN, Jennifer, "Preparing Before Your Surgery: Lifestyle Changes Before You Have Surgery," *About.com*, February 18, 2011, http://surgery.about.com/od/beforesurgery/ss/BeforeYourSurg_2.htm.

[34] Roizen, M.D, Michael F. and Oz, M.D., Mehmet C., *You The Smart Patient: An Insider's Handbook for Getting the Best Treatment*, (Free Press, 2006), 314-315.

[35] U.S. Department of Justice Drug Enforcement Administration, Office of Diversion Control, Controlled Substance Schedules, http://www.deadiversion.usdoj.gov/schedules/index.html.

[36] American Hospital Association, "Fast Facts on US Hospitals," January 3, 2013, *AHA.org*, http://www.aha.org/research/rc/stat-studies/fast-facts.shtml.

[37] The Advisory Board Company, "Ambulatory surgery centers may soon outnumber hospitals," *The Daily Briefing*, January 31, 2013, http://www.advisory.com/Daily-Briefing/2013/01/31/Ambulatory-surgery-centers-may-soon-outnumber-hospitals.

[38] New York State Bar Association, "Health Care Proxy: Appointing Your Health Care Agent in New York State," *nysba.org*, July, 2007, http://www.nysba.org/WorkArea/DownloadAsset.aspx?id=26503.

[39] The American Bar Association, "Giving Someone A Power of Attorney For Your Health Care: A Guide With An Easy-To-Use, Legal Form For All Adults," americanbar.org, 2011, http://www.americanbar.org/content/dam/aba/uncategorized/2011/2011_aging_hcdec_univh cpaform.authcheckdam.pdf.

[40] Illinois Department on Aging Advance Directives, "Illinois Statutory Short Form Power of Attorney For Health Care," *State.il.us*, http://www.state.il.us/aging/1news_pubs/publications/poa_healthcare.pdf.

[41] Toler, Alice, "Seasonal Affective Disorder: Home Remedies for the Winter Blues," *Catalyst Magazine*, February 2013, 18.

[42] Motz, Julie, *Hands of Life*, Bantam Books, New York, 1998.

[43] Brown, Chip, "The Experiments of Dr. Oz," *New York Times*, July 30, 1995, http://www.nytimes.com/1995/07/30/magazine/the-experiments-of-dr-oz.html.

[44] Hartford Hospital, Integrative Medicine, Outcomes, http://www.harthosp.org/integrativemed/outcomes/default.aspx#outcome6.

[45] "Therapeutic Touch," NYU Langone Medical Center, http://integrativehealth.med.nyu.edu/patient-care-partner-services/modalities-services/therapeutic-touch (accessed August 12, 2013).

[46] Brown, Chip, "The Experiments of Dr. Oz," *New York Times*, July 30, 1995, http://www.nytimes.com/1995/07/30/magazine/the-experiments-of-dr-oz.html.

[47] Mind-Body Bedside Patient Program, NYU Langone Medical Center, http://integrativehealth.med.nyu.edu/patient-and-care-partner-services/mind-body-patient-bedside-program.

[48] Riggio, Ph.D., Ronald E. and Stevenson, Sarah "There's Magic In Your Smile: How Smiling Affects Your Brain," *PsychologyToday.com*, June 25, 2012, http://www.psychologytoday.com/blog/cutting-edge-leadership/201206/there-s-magic-in-your-smile.

[49] "Saccharomyces Boulardii Overview Information," *WebMD.com*, http://www.webmd.com/vitamins-supplements/ingredientmono-332-saccharomyces%20boulardii.aspx?activeIngredientId=332&activeIngredientName= saccharomyces%20boulardii.

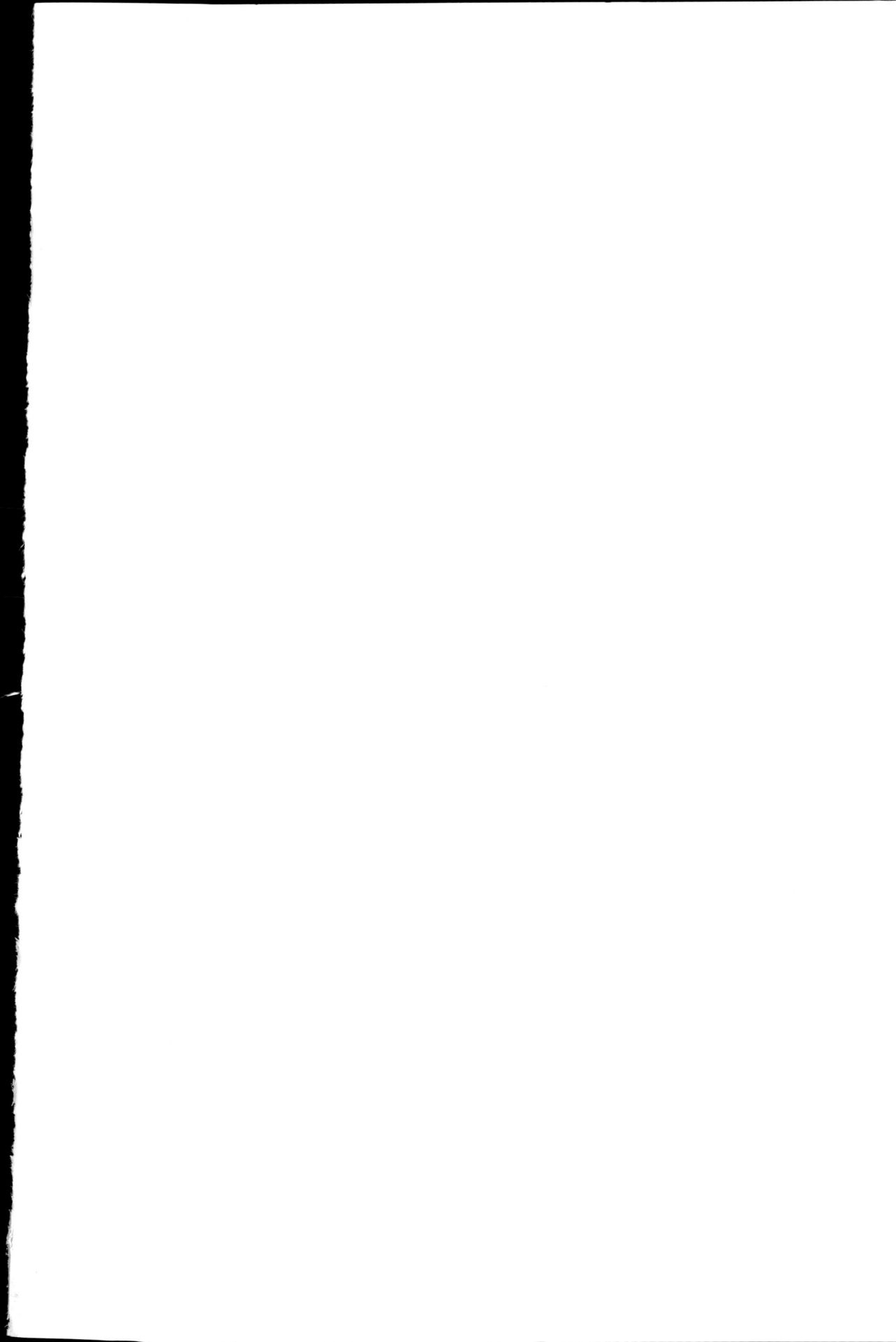

www.ingramcontent.com/pod-product-compliance
Lightning Source LLC
Chambersburg PA
CBHW062030210326
41519CB00061B/7428